Sexually Compulsive Behavior: Hypersexuality

Guest Editors

MARK F. SCHWARTZ, ScD
FRED S. BERLIN, MD, PhD

PSYCHIATRIC CLINICS OF NORTH AMERICA

www.psych.theclinics.com

December 2008 • Volume 31 • Number 4

SAUNDERS an imprint of ELSEVIER, Inc.

W.B. SAUNDERS COMPANY
A Division of Elsevier Inc.

1600 John F. Kennedy Boulevard • Suite 1800 • Philadelphia, PA 19103-2899

http://www.theclinics.com

PSYCHIATRIC CLINICS OF NORTH AMERICA Volume 31, Number 4
December 2008 ISSN 0193-953X, ISBN-13: 978-1-4160-6389-6, ISBN-10: 1-4160-6389-7

Editor: Sarah E. Barth
Developmental Editor: Donald Mumford

Psychiatric Clinics of North America (ISSN 0193-953X) is published quarterly by Elsevier Inc., 360 Park Av South, New York, NY 10010-1710. Months of issue are March, June, September, and December. Business Editorial Offices: 1600 John F. Kennedy Blvd., Suite 1800, Philadelphia, PA 19103-2899. Customer Servi Office: 6277 Sea Harbor Drive, Orlando, FL 32887-4800 Periodicals postage paid at New York, NY and addi tional mailing offices. Subscription prices are $230.00 per year (US individuals), $398.00 per year (US institu- tions), $116.00 per year (US students/residents), $275.00 per year (Canadian individuals), $495.00 per year (Canadian Institutions), $342.00 per year (foreign individuals), $495.00 per year (foreign institutions), and $171.00 per year (international & Canadian students/residents). Foreign air speed delivery is included in all *Clinics*' subscription prices. All prices are subject to change without notice. **POSTMASTER:** Send address changes to *Psychiatric Clinics of North America*, Elsevier Periodicals Customer Service, 11830 Westline Indus- trial Drive, St. Louis, MO 63146. Customer Service: 1-800-654-2452 (US). From outside the United States, call 1-314-453-7041. Fax: 1-314-453-5170. E-mail: JournalsCustomerServiceusa@elsevier.com (for print support) and JournalsOnlineSupport-usa@elsevier.com (for online support).

Reprints. For copies of 100 or more, of articles in this publication, please contact the Commercial Reprints Department, Elsevier Inc., 360 Park Avenue South, New York, New York 10010-1710. Tel.: (212) 633-3813, Fax: (212) 462-1935, E-mail: reprints@elsevier.com.

Psychiatric Clinics of North America is covered in *MEDLINE/PubMed (Index Medicus)*, *Current Contents/Social and Behavioral Sciences, Social Science Citation Index, Embase/Excerpta Medica,* and PsycINFO.

Printed in the United States of America.

Contributors

GUEST EDITORS

MARK F. SCHWARTZ, ScD
Assistant Professor of Psychiatry and Neurology, Saint Louis University, St. Louis; and Clinical Director, Castlewood Treatment Center, Ballwin, Missouri

FRED S. BERLIN, MD, PhD
Associate Professor, Department of Psychiatry and Behavioral Sciences, The Johns Hopkins University School of Medicine, Baltimore, Maryland

AUTHORS

GENE G. ABEL, MD
Professor of Clinical Psychiatry, Emory University School of Medicine; Professor of Clinical Psychiatry, Morehouse School of Medicine; Behavioral Medicine Institute of Atlanta; and President, Abel Screening, Inc., Atlanta, Georgia

JOHN BANCROFT, MD
Senior Research Fellow (formerly Director), The Kinsey Institute for Research in Sex, Gender and Reproduction, Indiana University, Bloomington, Indiana; and Barnhurst, Horspath, Oxfordshire, United Kingdom

FRED S. BERLIN, MD, PhD
Associate Professor, Department of Psychiatry and Behavioral Sciences, The Johns Hopkins University School of Medicine, Baltimore, Maryland

DONALD W. BLACK, MD
Professor of Psychiatry, Department of Psychiatry, University of Iowa Roy J. and Lucille A. Carver College of Medicine, Iowa City, Iowa

VICTORIA L. CODISPOTI, MD, D-FAPA
Private Practice of Forensic Psychiatry, Salem, Illinois

LATRICIA COFFEY, MD
Morehouse School of Medicine; and Laurel Heights Hospital, Atlanta, Georgia

JAMES GERBER, PhD
Castlewood Treatment Center, Ballwin, Missouri

JOHN M. KUZMA, MD
HealthPartners Regions Behavioral Health, St. Paul, Minnesota

LIAM E. MARSHALL, MA
Senior Therapist and Research Manager, Rockwood Psychological Services, Kingston, Ontario, Canada

WILLIAM L. MARSHALL, OC, PhD, FRSC
Director, Rockwood Psychological Services; and Professor Emeritus, Department of Psychology, Queen's University, Kingston, Ontario, Canada

MATT D. O'BRIEN, MSc
Therapist, Rockwood Psychological Services, Kingston, Ontario, Canada

CANDICE A. OSBORN, MA, LPC
Behavioral Medicine Institute of Atlanta, Atlanta, Georgia

COLIN A. ROSS, MD
President, The Colin A. Ross Institute for Psychological Trauma, Richardson, Texas

MARK F. SCHWARTZ, ScD
Assistant Professor of Psychiatry and Neurology, Saint Louis University, St. Louis; and Clinical Director, Castlewood Treatment Center, Ballwin, Missouri

GERRIS A. SERRAN, PhD
Clinical Director Prison Programs, Rockwood Psychological Services, Kingston, Ontario, Canada

STEPHEN SOUTHERN, EdD
Professor and Chair, Department of Psychology, Mississippi College, Clinton, Mississippi

DAN J. STEIN, MD, PhD
Professor of Psychiatry,University of Cape Town, Cape Town, South Africa; and Professor of Psychiatry, Mt. Sinai School of Medicine, New York

MARTHA TURNER, MD
Private Practice, Bryn Mawr, Pennsylvania

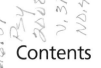

Contents

Highly pernicious events can result in a variety of severe adult psychiatric manifestations, including pedophilia in select individuals with a history of prior "at-risk factors." Influences such as social isolation can either increase or decrease the outcome. This article reviews some of the other sequential developmental factors that might contribute to sexual compulsivity in such biographies, including temperament, early attachment, family influences, trauma re-enactments, affect dysregulation, social isolation, vandalized love maps, self-formation, sexualization in families, and addictive cycles.

Patients with clinically excessive sexual thoughts or behaviors have been categorized as suffering from a compulsive, impulsive, or addictive sexual disorder. Similar considerations apply to a range of other impulse control disorders, such as excessive gambling. We have elsewhere proposed that in such conditions, phenomenological and psychobiological considerations suggest that key components include affective dysregulation, behavioral addiction, and cognitive dyscontrol. We argue here that there are advantages to using terms (such as hypersexual disorder) that go beyond the compulsive-impulsive-addictive delineation, and we advocate that additional work to characterize the phenomenology and psychobiology of hypersexual disorder and other conditions characterized by affective dysregulation, behavioral addiction, and cognitive dyscontrol be undertaken in the hope it will lead to improved assessment and management.

Explaining how and why sexual behavior gets out of control is fundamentally important to the advancement of effective treatments. In this article,

THE CLINICS ARE NOW AVAILABLE ONLINE!

Access your subscription at:
www.theclinics.com

Preface

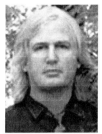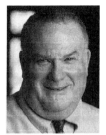

Mark F. Schwartz, ScD   Fred S. Berlin, MD, PhD
Guest Editors

Psychiatric diagnoses constitute a short-hand way of conveying information—information that may assist in guiding treatment and helping patients. Historically, as time has passed and new knowledge emerged, professional and societal ways of appreciating mental and behavioral capacities and impairments have changed. The alcoholic, once believed to be morally corrupt, is now more often and correctly appreciated as a human being in need of professional assistance. Many people previously believed to be lazy are now more often correctly identified as victims of clinical depression.

With respect to sexual issues, in the 1970s there seems to have been a virtual epidemic of rapid ejaculation and female anorgasmia, possibly resulting from strict, shame-based sexual prohibitions during childhood. As time passed, however, and patients gained greater knowledge about what constituted a normal and healthy sexual response, feelings of shame declined and the incidence of such cases decreased dramatically. The 1980s brought an increased recognition of etiologic and psychologic problems related to the violence of rape and to the potential trauma of incest. At the same time there was an increased focus on dysfunctions of sexual desire and arousal, and an increased focus on pedophilia and its associated sequelae. In the 1990s, because of the widespread use of computers and access to the Internet, a new venue emerged among both males and females for the expression of problems related to hypersexuality, paraphilias, cybersex, so-called "sexual addiction," and what has often seemed to be out-of-control sexual behavior. Historically, as new problems have been identified, the following decades have then been filled with advances in research, scientific publications, books, theories, concepts, and treatments, many of which have withstood the test of time.

This issue is one of the first to bring together some of the most outstanding specialists in the field of what some are now calling hypersexual behaviors, to share theoretically based research and to try to work through the related conceptual issues. In doing so, various authors have considered developmental (Schwartz), epidemiologic (Kuzma and Black), sexual arousal (Abel, Coffey, & Osborn), conceptual (Bancroft), biologic (Berlin), and pharmacologic (Codispodi) issues related to the concept of human hypersexuality. At the same time potentially new syndromes related to women (Turner),

Psychiatr Clin N Am 31 (2008) xi–xii
doi:10.1016/j.psc.2008.08.001   **psych.theclinics.com**

adolescents (Gerber), or dissociative clients (Ross) have been introduced. The use of computers for sexual purposes, with a special emphasis on treatment (Marshall and colleagues) has also been reviewed.

The intended result has been an integration of the current state of this young field, designed to help guide clinicians through the often bewildering and baffling maze of these difficult-to-treat conditions. The bases of sexual desire and arousal and of normal and pathologic sexual behaviors have been explored in depth. Special consideration has been given to trying to clarify the current mixed diagnostic plethora of terms (such as impulsive, compulsive, dissociative, addictive, hypersexual, and intimacy- and attachment-related disorders), with the additional goal of trying to assist in bringing greater clarity for the next edition of the *Diagnostic and Statistical Manual of Mental Disorders*.

It seems likely that new psychiatric concepts will continue to emerge and evolve over time. Those of us who have devoted our lives to understanding and treating patients afflicted with psychiatric illnesses must change and evolve too. We cannot succeed without a reliable influx of new and credible evidence-based information and ideas. This issue strives to supply information about hypersexuality as an important contemporary psychiatric issue, while also serving as a useful guide for psychiatrists and other mental health professionals who may be interested in this developing multidiscipline.

Mark F. Schwartz, ScD
Clinical Director
Castlewood Treatment Center
800 Holland Road
Ballwin, MO 63021, USA

Fred S. Berlin, MD, PhD
Associate Professor
Johns Hopkins University
104 East Biddle Street
Baltimore, MD 21202, USA

E-mail addresses:
mfs96@aol.com (M.F. Schwartz)
fredsberlinmd@comcast.net (F.S. Berlin)

Developmental Psychopathological Perspectives on Sexually Compulsive Behavior

Mark F. Schwartz, ScD

KEYWORDS

- Trauma • Sexually compulsive behavior
- Hyposexuality • Hypersexuality

The developmental factors that contribute to sexually compulsive behavior, para-philias, and sex offender behavior have been poorly delineated,[1] and that which has been written on the subject is stuck in a conceptual quagmire. Marshall[2] stated, "It is important to note that our theory suggests that a failure to attain intimacy in relation-ships is but one aspect of the development and maintenance of sexual deviance. We have at other times, pointed to sociocultural factors,[3] the role of pornography,[4] and biological processes and interaction as well as conditioning[5] and developmental ex-periences."[6] In other words, many factors may contribute, depending on the clients.

How best to embrace and incorporate these factors into a successful treatment ap-proach? A developmental psychopathological perspective may provide the answer. It is a robust conceptual frame that departs from such traditional models of unidimen-sional static "causes" of a disorder[7] and instead postulates a developmental trajec-tory for a symptom in the evolutionary context of the individual attempting to adapt.[8] Critical life events precipitate other positive or negative life experiences or cir-cumstances and then mitigate them, thereby increasing or decreasing the resulting degree of disability and the likelihood of symptom emergence. Adaptation continually unfolds within an ever-changing context, which allows for developmental deviation or amelioration of an ontogenetic process.[9]

Maladaptation can result from different developmental pathways, which are proba-bilistically related to disturbance. Individuals who begin on similar paths may diverge and manifest different symptoms of psychopathology. Despite marked initial devia-tion, the capacity to rebound is mediated by prior adaptation and evolves over time within the total framework of developmental influence. To treat a client according to

Castlewood Treatment Center, 800 Holland Road, Ballwin, MO 63021, USA
E-mail address: mfs96@aol.com

Psychiatr Clin N Am 31 (2008) 567–586
doi:10.1016/j.psc.2008.07.002
0193-953X/08/$ – see front matter © 2008 Elsevier Inc. All rights reserved.

this model, the clinician must endeavor to construct or reconstruct all contributing biologic, psychological, and social trends from an individual's past and present to understand coalescence into the individual's current functioning.

To illustrate, I was recently involved in a court case in which 20 men came forward after public disclosure that a priest had molested children in their church for many years. As boys, they had known one another and had witnessed their friends being molested at or near puberty. None of the boys had ever been to a mental health care professional. All 20 men were severely impaired with Axis I and Axis II diagnoses, but none had attributed his psychiatric symptoms to the repeated molestations until they heard the newscast. All the men had relational and sexual difficulties that included pedophilia,[2] ego dystonic homosexuality (2), hyposexuality (8), hypersexuality (6), and asexuality (2).[10] Viewed through this conceptual lens, one could conclude that a virulent event, such as molestation by a priest, is of such magnitude that it injures almost everyone, but the manifestation of that injury is variable and related to a multitude of other factors. We do not know, for instance, how many men were molested but did not come forth or whether they all have such severe symptoms.

In the backgrounds of these men, most showed social isolation and serious problems in relating to others. More than 90% had no friends. Only 20% of this sample thought that their parents treated them well. None had difficulties with the law beyond drug abuse or alcohol-related offenses. My search for other contributing influences included a review of the empirical literature. Abel and colleagues[11] noted that 58.4% of sex offenders reported onset of their deviant sexual arousal before age 18. Other factors found to be predictive of sexual deviation have included a history of parental conflict, poor parental supervision, and lack of affection by the mothers.[12] Each of these boys had difficulty transitioning through adolescence and forming adult relationships and—to different degrees—a combination of these risk factors.

This case illustrates abuse from clergy as one example of a highly pernicious event that results in a variety of severe adult psychiatric manifestations, including pedophilia in select individuals with a history of prior "at-risk factors." The case also shows that influences such as social isolation can either increase or decrease the outcome. This article reviews some of the other sequential developmental factors that might contribute to sexual compulsivity in such biographies, including temperament, early attachment, family influences, trauma re-enactments, affect dysregulation, social isolation, vandalized love maps, self-formation, sexualization in families, and addictive cycles.

TEMPERAMENT AND SEXUAL COMPULSIVITY

Cloninger and colleagues[13] suggested that the relay race of developmental influences begins with temperament. They stated that temperament consists of autonomic impulses in response to basic associative stimuli that give rise to primary emotions such as fear, anger, disgust, and determination. Four independent inherent dimensions that emanate from discernible brain systems have been distinguished: harm avoidance (anxiety proneness, risk taking), novelty seeking (impulsiveness and rigidity), reward dependency (approval seeking and aloofness), and persistence (determination and fixedness). Cloninger and colleagues[13] correlated these temperaments with dimensions of character in a step-wise fashion.

Cloninger's system overlaps with the longitudinal data of Caspi and colleagues[14], in which they isolated temperament patterns of 3-year-old children as (1) uncontrolled, (2) inhibited, or (3) well-adjusted. They followed the children longitudinally to discover that "uncontrolled" children externalized their problems at age 10 and, at a later age, scored low on constraint. These children described themselves as reckless and careless and said they enjoyed dangerous activities. At age 18, the "inhibited" children were shy, fearful, and ill at ease socially. These temperaments are predictive of the compulsive style (inhibited) of the acting-in individual and the impulsive style (uncontrolled) of acting-out clients as sexual compulsives. In Cloninger's typology, if it is likely that the individual predisposed to be out of control sexually is either impulsive (novelty seeking) or compulsive (persistence) at an early age,[11] both "uncontrolled" and "inhibited" fit the latter profile of select adolescent sexual compulsives.[15] Disinhibition caused by alcohol, drugs, or anger has been noted commonly in individuals who are sexually out of control.[16] For some individuals, sexually out-of-control behavior is part of general antisocial tendencies,[17] along with nonconformity and impulsivity.[18] Although little research currently exists on the topic, it is likely that temperament factors are important in distinguishing which at-risk individuals eventually will act out sexually and the ways in which they will act out. Areas that need study include the identifying consequences of early impulsivity and compulsivity, determining which individuals within these categories are at risk for acting in or acting out, determining which individuals are likely to be socially inhibited, and identifying individuals at risk for lack of empathy. Caspi's work suggested that these characteristics can be measured reliably by age 3. It is likely that temperament contributes to some percentage of the variance that explains how individuals with similar trauma may react differently.

ATTACHMENT AND SEXUALLY COMPULSIVE BEHAVIOR

Sexually compulsive behavior can be understood best under the superordinate category of courtship disorder[19] or as a "disorder of bonding or intimacy."[20] Fehrenbach and Monastersky[21] found that 65% of 305 juvenile sex offenders showed significant signs of social isolation and had serious problems relating to others. Thirty-two percent had no friends, and 34% were more isolated than nonsexual adolescent offenders who were chronically violent. Intimacy disorders have three common deficits:[22] (1) impaired sense of self, (2) difficulty with affect regulation, and (3) impairment in ability to turn to others for comfort and safety. Effective treatment of hypersexualities often requires changes in each of these areas. Each of these subtopics is discussed briefly.

Impaired Sense of Self

In his review of the development of the brain and origin of self, Schore[23] articulated the initial role of the mother-child dyad elegantly:

> "The child's first relationship acts as a template and it molds the individual's capacities to enter into all emotional relationships. Development essentially represents a number of sequentially mutually driven infant-care-giver processes that occur in a continuous dialectic between the maturing organism and the changing environment. It now appears that affect is what is actually transacted within the mother-infant dyad, and the highly efficient system of emotional connection is essentially nonverbal."

The mother's attunement to the child facilitates the experience-dependent maturation of the neurologic hard wiring of the child's brain—hierarchically from the lower limbic emotional structures through the midbrain and up to other cortical structures—during this early critical period.[24] Therapists are discovering that strong affect is the window into "deep structure" in which core beliefs (schema) and unconscious internal working models shape the love maps during the first 10 years of life.[25,26] More attention is currently being paid to the attachment between infants and caretakers in the first years of life, mostly stimulated by the original writings of John Bowlby.[26]

Table 1 includes a summary of empirically established attachment patterns. A secure attachment in these early years provides a child with the security needed to confidently explore the environment, develop feelings of empathy for others,[27] have positive self-esteem, and, ultimately, have better quality adult love relationships, friendships, and acquaintanceships.[28] Attachment problems can become more likely when there is (1) disruption in which the attachment figure is perceived as unloving (depressed mothers), (2) parental abuse or the attachment figure is seen as the source of danger and safety, (3) a subjective sense of feeling abandoned by the attachment figure, particularly at a time of crisis, and (4) loss of an attachment figure by death or injury.[27] Individuals adapt to such attachment trauma either by dismissing the need for attachment and potentially any available connection (avoidants) or by becoming "preoccupied" with their hunger for love but being anxious about rejection, as occurs frequently with so called "sex addicts." Such individuals are starving for love but confuse genital sexuality with feelings of loneliness and disconnection. The "disorganized" style combines both strategies and is the prototype of "intimacy disorder" in our culture.

Inadequate early attachment bonds are highly predictive of later relationship distress. Individuals rated as "anxious/ambivalent" are starving and fearful of close relationships, whereas "avoidant" children later often report never having been in love or never having experienced strong feelings of love.[29] Sexuality is generally a manifestation of attachment difficulties, so the "preoccupied" individual can have anonymous sex with multiple individuals in an evening without feeling sated. The "avoidant"

Table 1
Summary of attachment patterns

Child	Adult
Secure	Secure
• Seeks comfort	• Coherence
• Caregiver is a secure base relieved upon return of mom; seeks comfort, feels comforted, resumes play; relaxes completely in mother's arms, allows full embrace, goes back to play	• Consistency • Collaboration
Avoidant	Dismissing
• Minimizes distress; avoids contact	• Idealization with discrepancies
• It is as if the mother has not re-entered the room; Stroufe showed elevated heart rate that does not decline with mother's return	• Insistence on inability to recall childhood
	• Derogating dismissal (rarely: fear of loss of child through death)
Resistant/Ambivalent	Preoccupied
• Heightens distress—ambivalent	• Involves preoccupying anger
• Seeks contact but is whiney, resistant, ambivalent to contact (approach/avoidance)	• Passivity/vagueness in discourse
Disorganized	Unresolved/Disorganized
• Contradictory behaviors	• States of mind with respect to experiences of loss and responses to abuse

person goes out with prostitutes and has mechanical sex without affection or emotional connection.[30] Of recent interest are individuals assessed with disorganized attachment.[31] Researchers originally identified children who in the "strange situation" at 18 months of age approached and avoided the returning parent and often appeared dazed, confused, and apprehensive. The researchers hypothesized that this behavior is related to the parent's struggle with unresolved trauma of his or her own. Ogawa and colleagues[32] also identified a link between disorganized attachment during the child's first 29 months and adult dissociation. Disorganized individuals in adulthood are described by themselves and friends as somewhat introverted, cold, and emotionally void;[32] they do not know how to turn to others for help. They lack a "secure base."

The importance of using the lens of attachment theory is that sexual disorders can be understood as difficulties with pair-bonding, courtship, attraction, love, affection, and intimacy. Without adequate parenting, a child grapples with "increased" appetite for nurturing and caretaking while simultaneously adapting by becoming dismissive of such needs, with expectations of being hurt, disappointed, and abandoned. In this way, needs themselves are "dangerous" and associated with fear. The solution to needing and fearing is paraphilia. A person becomes aroused by pictures and objects rather than people—a fetish can distance and provide a ritualistic illusion of control in what would otherwise be a terrifying situation. The object does not abandon or hurt and provides comfort. Preoccupied individuals undoubtedly turn to more and more sex to fill the needs for caretaking, whereas avoidant individuals use sexual activity to be alone and disconnect but still feel alive and experience some affective respite from emptiness through the intense release.

When individuals experience misattunement with their caretakers during infancy, they fail to establish a secure attachment and the feelings internally of being loveable and entitled to job and connection with others. Injury to this attachment system impairs their ability to "metabolize" stress, because humans need to talk to others and receive comfort when overwhelmed. When there is misattunement with the caretaker, children actively anticipate their mother's reaction and inhibit or minimize their internal experience of "needing," which results in avoidance of intimacy. Other children amplify or maximize awareness and the expression of attachment, feeling, and needs in response to periodically getting their needs met. Children hyperactivate their attachment system to capture their mother's unpredictable attention.

Like these infants, sexually compulsive individuals actively maintain the "rules of attachment" laid down in infancy. Some deny their unmet emotional needs by distracting themselves with sexual obsessions. Others are consumed with doubt of the partner's love and require sex as a constant reassurance of being loveable. Their sexual behavior ultimately serves the function of preserving unaltered internal working models of attachment. To change these cemented patterns, the primary focus of treatment needs to be on facilitating the development of secure attachment with self and others, which begins with an attuned relationship with the therapist. The therapist who focuses on changing the internal working model is maximally effective.

Attachment and Self Systems

Disorganized attachment results in individuals who turn to paraphilia as an active survival strategy to cope with the inability to articulate internal states and turn to other people for comfort. Clients unconsciously deploy their attention to sex to shore up and justify pre-existing expectations of unresponsive and unpredictable caring. Individuals actively use paraphilia to avoid anticipated rejection in intimate relations. The result of disorganized attachment is that it leads to the development of segregated, dissociated internal working models of self and the attachment figure. The individual states, "I don't know who I am," "I feel like an imposter," or "I'm really bad but pretend to be good." This is starkly exemplified by the priest who has been a "devoted servant of God" but molests children or has chronic affairs with church wives or the family man who has routine homosexual liaisons or engages repetitively in "sexually addictive" forms of acting out. Similar to the childhood experience of the mother who was both kind and mean, the person may perceive closeness with all potential partners as necessary and distressing, which leads to monumental courtship ambivalence and numbing of experiences of affection.

Within the developmental model of affectional systems, critical capacities must be assimilated or symptoms may emerge. These skills include affect regulation, social skills, and perceived efficacy in attempting to negotiate social relationships, empathy and compassion for others, and capacity for accurate attunement regarding cues from others. These structural capacities make up the stage on which psychological drama unfolds.[33] These are the targets of developmentally based psychotherapies. Child abuse and neglect are common factors in the histories of individuals who manifest hypo- and hypersexualities. It is critical to dissect the structural deficits that occur with abuse and neglect and use cognitive-affective-behavioral therapies for developmental repair.

At the core of one's capacity to bond are self-empathy and the capacity for self-care. In the absence of alternative validating caretakers, the individual does not internalize a caring relationship with self. A child who is rejected or abandoned tends to develop negative core schemas or beliefs about self. Accompanying modes of processing and organizing information (including affects) unfold such that these beliefs become self-perpetuating. These modes ultimately organize an individual's range and type of interactions, which constrains possibilities for new learning with respect to intimacy. Such difficulties have caused some to describe sex offenders as "fixated," that is, structurally stuck at child and adolescent stages of development and fearful of adult relationships and burdens.

The self comes to exist in the context of others, within an aggregation of experiences of the self in relationship. Invariant aspects of the self and others in relationships are abstracted into what Bowlby called "internal representational models." New experiences are then absorbed into earlier representations, creating and maintaining an individual who is distinct from others. The internal working models of sexually compulsive individuals are filled with self-hatred and the need to compensate by pretending to be powerful, effective, or competent. This imposter imbalance creates anxiety, and eventually the sexual behavior allows them the relief of being caught and punished.

The individual also creates self functions, which are tools to negotiate interactions with others, manage the intensity of the experience, and balance inner and outer experiences. Self functions navigate the balance between their old and new experiences by means of moderating intense feelings. Examples of self functions include social skills, appropriate affects with others, social anxiety, listening abilities, anger management problem solving, and tolerance empathy, all of which sexually compulsive individuals often find difficult. Availability of self-efficacy determines behavioral manifestations of alternating degrees of closeness and distance. When the balance of closeness and distance is dysfunctional rather than adaptive, intimacy disorders emerge.

One type of intimacy disorder originates when a child experiences a disorganized attachment.[34,35] An infant becomes highly sensitized to soothing the caretaker, presumably to exert control and self-protection. The cost of surviving is giving up the development and differentiation of an autonomous self, which requires sufficient safety to individuate. The individual then attempts to create safety and consistency in malad-aptive ways (ie, distorted survival strategies). In this intimacy dysfunction, an individual repeatedly finds individuals who need care to construct an illusion of safety and con-trol. They become an extension of their partner's identity, and their boundaries be-come blurred such that it feels as if the other is vital to the self's survival. They simultaneously experience a need to merge like a child to a caretaker and a need to run for fear of being engulfed or abandoned. They also experience ambivalence re-lated to the need to use others for self-soothing versus being independent. If sexuality has been injured in its unfolding through association with violence or loss of control, ambivalence extends more profoundly into the closeness/distance continuum. This ambivalence can be played out in myriad destructive ways, ranging from repetitive af-fairs to low sexual drive.

Deficits in the first year of life typically lead to self-cohesion difficulties and leave the individual vulnerable to fragmentation. Epstein[36] suggested that the result of internal self-fragmentation is the creation, metaphorically speaking, of "black holes that absorb fear and create the defensive posture of the isolated self unable to make satisfying contact with oneself or others." Without basic integration, the individual experiences one's identity as many "selves" or feels like an imposter because of in-herent experience of contradiction. Each of these "selves" has the capacity to pro-duce behavior and has impulses for action. One system can be cut off from another, leading to unconscious motives for behavior. This fragmentation may explain why some individuals can find young children sexually arousing (ie, a part of self with a developmental age of 6–10 takes executive control but has the sexual arousal of an adult). Where there is extreme internal encapsulation, a person can act with seeming integrity (such as a member of the clergy or the principal of a school), have multiple sexual partners or molest a child, lie to others, and seem sincere while actually not ex-periencing conflict or the implied contradiction. The mechanism of dissociation allows for the apparent anomaly in which "good people do bad things." This explanation of deviant sexual arousal patterns is consistent with the repeated findings of early ne-glect and abuse in the biography of sexual offenders.[37] In more extreme cases with early parental deprivation, sexual acting out can become more violent and manifest as revenge.[38]

During the second and third years of life, self-constancy is established. A child de-velops tolerance for separation and the capacity for self-soothing. He or she begins to internalize the belief in "being loved and valued" and does not need constant reassur-ance. Children form a positive self-object,[39] which allows them to experience a schema internally for being cared for in the absence of the caretaker. For example, children raised in state institutions in Romania and adopted in the United States may need to be told "I love you" by their caretaker 100 times a day because they do not have an internal structure to retain the belief.[40] In committed relationships, such indi-viduals may desire sex constantly to feel desired or may need to seduce or flirt com-pulsively to feel desirable.

By 4 years of age, a child develops self-agency or the ability to operate in the world and actively create or elicit responses from others. A child develops a lexicon for affect and forms a framework for self-efficacy and mastery. The result of the healthy devel-opment of self-cohesion, self-constancy, and self-agency is self-esteem. Positive af-fect becomes integrated with self-representation. Individuals with intimacy disorders may lack a positive self-object and require others' constant mirroring to maintain their sense of self. They become highly suggestible and susceptible to influence. They chronically lack self-esteem and engage in human "doing" rather than "being," be-cause they experience themselves as being only as good as their last response.

Men who have anonymous sex with multiple partners in a night may verbalize that they "feel only as good as their last trick." This is similar to individuals driven to make one business deal after another—at great cost to their family life—to attain more money, more status, or other illusions of safety.

The love map, which organizes the self-functions and facilitates relational choices, is structured by 5 or 6 years of age. Perceptions of what is attractive in oneself and one's potential partners are organized in the care of the love map. Persons with vandalized love maps maintain a "confirming bias" by selective interaction with others in the environment. They choose relations that fit the exiting core schemata and avoid or devalue relations that might refute central beliefs and affects of the schemata. In this manner, an individual with intimacy disorder is held captive by the damaged love map until new learning can occur.

Affect Dysregulation

Abused children encounter substantial difficulty in accomplishing the developmental task of acquiring an effective strategy for regulation of their emotions within their relationship with caretakers,[41] which contributes to further social rejection. Learning to turn to people as a source of comfort is essential for metabolizing toxic negative emotions, and fearing close relationships leaves individuals vulnerable to alternative solutions, such as public exposure or fetishes. Some individuals, however, seem to be "saved" by novel experiences with a loving caretaker, teacher, friend, girlfriend, or therapist. During the young adolescent years, there are rehearsals of courtship proceptive behavior,[42] such as touching, kissing, holding hands, and so on. Boys who fall behind with courtship develop social anxieties and fears that cause them to fall further behind. They often turn to pornography, which becomes a reservoir of deviant arousal conditioning at a critical period when they are flooded with testicular androgens. Girls also may visit sexual Internet sites or chat rooms, which likewise introduce opportunities for deviant experiences to experientially vulnerable and naïve individuals (see the article by Martha Turner in this issue).

Sroufe[35] found that avoidantly attached boys were more likely to bully, lie, cheat, destroy things, brag, act cruelly, disrupt the class, swear, tease, threaten, argue, and throw temper tantrums, whereas girls were more likely to become depressed and blame themselves. The same early deprivation leads to more acting out and aggression in boys, which is likely the reason that boys are much more inclined to meld aggression with sexual behavior as a solution to affect dysregulation. Herman[43] observed that abused children develop maladaptive self-regulatory mechanisms. "Abused children discover they can produce release through emotions becoming dysregulated and the child is unable to find a consistent strategy for establishing comfort and security under stress. Such individuals become more likely to exhibit self-destructive behavior—acting in or acting out."

These same individuals are also impaired in their capacity to reflect on their own feelings and those of others.[44] They often seek chaotic relationships, recreating and re-enacting the familiar early rejections and frustrations in new formats with peers in school,[45] which likely is a way of dealing with autonomic dysregulation.[46] Purging, vomiting, compulsive sexual behavior, compulsive risk taking, gambling, and exposure to alcohol and drugs become vehicles with which abused children regulate their internal state. Abused and neglected children anticipate abandonment, rejection, unfairness, and conflict with caretakers and teachers, which then leads to powerful feelings of rage, anxiety, and helplessness. Unable to establish safety in or out of the home, they survive by suppressing affect and then are compulsively driven to activity for release. Acting out is often punished ostensibly for the "child's own good,"[47] which further suppresses rage and activates the search for additional tension-reducing activity. Tension reduction affords self-soothing, anesthesia from pain, and restoration of affective control, which increase the likelihood of repeating the behavior.

Suppression of affect seems to leak into somatic function,[48] which causes increased medical symptoms, and into somatic symptoms related to sexuality (more common in males) and eating disorders (more common in females). Individuals seems to interpret strong emotions as synonymous cognitively with a desire for compulsive acting out (ie, I'm lonely = I need sex; I'm frustrated = I need sex; I'm sad = I need a sexual partner). These releases are exacerbated by increased autonomic arousal.[49] Individuals may feel sad, angry, or lonely but within the context of alexithymia, they experience the affect as hypersexuality and may turn, for example, to Internet sexuality for hours, cementing the connection and habit. In this manner, the individuals discover that this behavior can be self-soothing; it becomes a habit and eventually part of their identity (ie, I am an "exhibitionist," a "pervert"). The relationship with an object makes them feel more like an object even as it further insulates them from anticipated or actual rejection from other people.

TRAUMA RE-ENACTMENTS

In the dissociative daze of childhood sexual abuse, children seek to repeat elements of a traumatic event or unresolved ambivalent attachment (ie, they do to others what was done to them).[44] Often they identify with the aggressor and display assaultive behavior or turn the anger inward and develop self-destructive strategies.

Having studied adaptations to severe stressors in childhood, Horowitz[50] suggested that the common "natural" result of severe trauma is repetition, which consists of flashbacks, intrusions, and re-enactment, until there is completion. If the stress response cycle is not completed successfully, erroneous schema become engraved into the internal working model of self. Relationships created by unresolved individuals are likely to re-enact by means of disguised repetitions, with accompanying numbing and intrusions, throughout their lives.[51] Dissociative defenses that result from trauma and disorganized attachment interfere with completion and mastery and "working through" the trauma. The result is that many victims of childhood abuse experience memory disturbances and are left to repeat the trauma in disguised form, unaware of its origin.[52] Compulsive re-enactment often includes "acting-in" compulsions, such as self-cutting or eating disorder, or "acting-out" compulsions, such as hypersexual acting out or destructive relationship re-enactments, such as picking alcoholic partners or entering battering relationships. These re-enactments can become addictive and serve as distractions from the internal emptiness and constriction and give the individual the illusion of temporary connectedness, power, control, and relief from loneliness and depression. This reliance is further potentiated by endorphin release,[53,54] extreme alterations in cortisol regulation, and dopamine release from the median emminance.

Serendipitously, the study of victims of sexual abuse has resulted in a new understanding of paraphilia and sexual compulsive behavior. Men and women who are sexually abused frequently present clinically with violent paraphilic sexual arousal and imagery, which is the result of "trauma bonding."[55] In trauma bonding, there is a pairing of sexual arousal with terror and violence at a critical stage in the child's development. Thereafter, there is a tendency to revisit the terror and high arousal, as if to master, complete, or comprehend it. Clinically, traumatized children tend to repeat violence in their play rehearsals, and molested children often act out the molestation in their doll play. The following excerpt is an example from one sexually abused client:

> *"After dad awakened the sexual awareness, I couldn't understand it. As I got older, it became more and more of a problem for me. I couldn't turn to you, you would blame me. So I turned to boys who would duplicate some of those feelings—of being cared for or loved. I knew I was fooling myself. I felt the emptiness I was left with after my liaisons with boys, but it was all I had. I was desperate to feel loved. I needed affection, even if it was pretend affection. My need for affection was so strong, I couldn't say no to many people. Even though it left me feeling miserable."*

Adults traumatized as children seem to be frozen at the point of trauma, acting out the violence repeatedly in their self-destructive decisions. Sexually abused women often engage in self-mutilation, a compulsive-ritualized self-destructive act, and describe their response as "an intensely pleasurable release" that helps them feel alive. Psychologically, there is an analgesic effect associated with the cutting and likely an opioid endorphin release centrally, which the individual experiences as pleasurable.[56] Cognitively, there is dissociation and depersonalization. Dissociation in this situation implies a numbing out, a disconnection of thoughts and feelings. During the trauma, an individual may feel as if she is leaving her body and becoming part of the wall or ceiling, which is a functional defense against the intolerable feelings of being in a body that is under assault. Thereafter, dissociation may serve as an automatic defense. Depersonalization in this context reflects that the individual has been treated like an object; thereafter she feels like an object and objectifies others. Because of the trauma bond, abuse survivors repetitively re-victimize themselves and can seem to invite chaos and crisis—in some cases not just out of familiarity and expectation but also, paradoxically, as a means of mastering the trauma. Masochistically, the emotional and physical pain may "feel good" and provide an escape from the numbness and emptiness that result from the dissociation and depersonalization.

Dissociation in males seems somewhat different than in females. Research on the effects of posttraumatic stress on monkeys suggests that similar stress has gender-specific effects, with males more dramatically manifesting the impact. Male monkeys tend to act out more, whereas females typically act in. An adult male monkey deprived of parenting in childhood often attacks other monkeys viciously, acting out of fear, hyperresponsivity, and consequent anger.[57] The female monkey in the same context, also hyperreactive, bites herself and develops catatonic symptoms.

Human females who have been victims of neglect and sexual or physical abuse often report that they do not feel entitled to express their pain and fear retribution if they show strong emotion. When in close proximity to a male, particularly in a potentially intimate interchange, they dissociate. During any kind of sexual contact, they "numb out," not thinking or feeling but instead locked in terror, feeling unentitled to say no. On the biofeedback machine, discussion of a sexual encounter is often associated with levels of anxiety sufficient to precipitate a panic attack. A common sexually compulsive posture on the part of some women in response to the terror is to allow a "seductive" part of their personality to "take control" of the situation. They maintain the illusion that they are in control of their sexual victimization "this time." Human males, on the other hand, are often unaware of their effective states, being so dissociated that they never register fear, anger, anxiety, or any emotion other than irritability. When they approach a fearful situation, they bypass all affect, and their ritualized behavior patterns become the sole automatic response to fear-related situations. Men typically oscillate between overcontrolled working, drinking, eating, or sex to being out of control to avoid encountering or remembering situations that are terrifying. The masculine counterpart in acting-in behavior consists of rigid rules and rituals to bind the anxiety and quell the fear that they have at an unconscious level.

Frederick and Luecke[58] asked mothers of 882 children who were not sexually abused and 276 mothers of children who were sexually molested to indicate the sexual behaviors shown by their children. Twenty-five behaviors were more prevalent in the sexually abused children. A high frequency of sexual behavior was related to more severe abuse, a greater number of perpetrators, and the use of force. Similarly, among 1000 women who presented to our sexual trauma program, 1 out of 5 reported sexually abusing, most commonly while babysitting, as an adolescent. The following is a description written by one client:

"There was a time at age 10 (right before I almost got beat to death and put into a foster home) that I was babysitting while my parents were out of town. I felt so lonely and scared. I had an empty funny feeling inside I had to fill—I didn't know what it was. I found myself in the room where my younger brother was asleep. He evidently was sleeping nude because I really don't remember taking his unders down. I touched him down there so we could 'fill each other.' I felt sick as I started doing this but kept on a couple of seconds more. He was asleep and looked so innocent that I really felt disgusted and I stopped. I got really sick and ran crying because I was so ashamed. I wonder if he remembers it. I'm sure he does.

"I did the same thing one time with my younger sister. My older sister had taught me how to masturbate when I was 5 so men wouldn't touch me. I was changing my younger sister's panties and when I pulled them up I guess I was 'triggered' into wanting to 'break' her in. (So she wouldn't hurt? Or to get her used to it? Or maybe I even wondered what my older sister had gotten out of touching me?) I touched her and realized I didn't like what I was doing. I felt sick in my stomach—guilty—ashamed, and sorry for what I had attempted to do—or had started to do. I never even thought these things again—ever—with any children.

"One day (at age 21?)…my mother lived across the street from me. She would ask my husband if I could go drinking with her so I could drive home and it was okay with him. I was over at her house. I always had a 'need' to be close to mommy and hoped there would be that one day she would hold and comfort me—and tell me she was so sorry for what happened to me. That day she said, 'Let's go lie down.' I said, 'OK!' (I remember thinking—I was going to take a nap with my mommy!)

"We were lying down. I had my clothes on. She was lying there with her eyes shut. I glanced down and saw she wasn't covered. She was either undressed or dressed very seductively. Her leg moved out a little (while she was sleeping?). All of a sudden I felt anger, a rage, and an overwhelming feeling I can't describe. I wanted to molest my mother. I wanted to do to her what had been done to me by my father and stepfather. She had allowed it to happen—she knew about it all along. I wanted to rape her. I reached over and put my hand on her crotch and started to put my finger in her. She squirmed with a moan of desire and I snapped into reality. I was overwhelmed with feelings of sickness in my stomach. I felt both shame and guilt—I don't know. I got sick and went home. It has never been mentioned again."

For individuals such as these, victim becoming victimizer can present more as a dissociative-like repetition of what was done to them rather than paraphilic sexual arousal. For some, this behavior eventually becomes part of deviant sexual arousal patterns.

A member of the clergy, who professes celibacy and chastity, spends hours on the Internet cruising pornography Web sites and masturbating while "cybering" with a teenage boy. He is a survivor of childhood sexual abuse, who is unaware of how he is re-enacting the trauma in this distorted attempt to reclaim lost youth. A woman who had a pregnancy out of wedlock gave up her infant for adoption when she was 16 years old. At age 35, after having another child, she becomes addicted to cybersex contacts in which she is treated badly, like a "dirty slut." Her behavior reveals the unfinished contradiction in her life: "I may look normal and good, but secretly I'm bad and sexuality is the source of my badness."

Heterosexual men who had repetitive preadolescent sexual contacts with a man may become involved in same-sex chat and masturbation on the Internet as a means of re-enacting the question, "Am I gay?" For some married persons, cybersex is an ideal mechanism for revenge or "payback." Compulsive cybersex users explained to their spouses when detected, "Somebody out there wants me if you don't" and "You spend too much money on what you want. I'm entitled to have my way." Some of the examples are so paradoxical they are easily viewed as perverse. An attorney in the midst of prosecuting sex offenders sits in his office and repeatedly masturbates while using his work computer. The father of three adolescent girls, whom he encourages to "just say no" to sex, retires to his study and solicits in a chat room a teenager for a sexual liaison. The "Dr. Jekyll and Mr. Hyde" quality of these transactions reflects the strength of dissociation in disconnecting parts of the self.

The survival strategy of dissociation evolves in childhood to manage disparate experiences, such as tolerating physical abuse at home, while maintaining capacities for socializing and learning at school. Dissociation, through the mechanism of encapsulation, helps an individual forget overwhelming childhood experiences, which are fragmented and stored in various parts of memory. These dissociated experiences eventually leak into consciousness as re-enactments, however. The woman who is unable to refuse any sexual advance and responds repeatedly to solicitations on the Internet cannot remember the incest from her childhood. Paradoxically, the compulsive re-enactment does not let her forget the abuse that is repeated almost daily through the computer usage. In compulsive sexual behavior, it is likely that an ego state has evolved to re-enact unfinished business, whereas the executive self parents, goes to work, or otherwise maintains a normal lifestyle.[59]

Compulsive sexual behavior also can function as a distraction from the burdensome consequences of selfhood, such as shame and perfectionism. Any tension-reducing event, such as bingeing or purging in bulimia, self-cutting, or compulsively masturbating to orgasm serves the function of narrowing the perceptual field to concrete events and refocusing the attention away from distressing cognition and affect. Masturbation during cybersex suppresses awareness and expression of emotion.

The body symbolizes the playing field for working through unsolvable life problems. One cybersex addict embraced the numbing, depersonalizing quality of his compulsive sexual behavior. He had sex with his brother's wife more than 20 years ago. His brother was killed in an accident 2 days after the affair. During therapy, he wondered if his brother committed suicide or, in a childlike ego state, he imagined he caused his brother's death. He took his brother's place by being immersed in affairs and becoming dead to the world. His compulsive sexual behavior ultimately became his dissociative effort at reconciling the unreconcilable: "My shameful out-of-control sex killed my brother" and "I can't tell anyone, but my illicit behavior will eventually cause me to get the punishment I deserve."

Compulsive sexual behavior can become a primary or exclusive means of sexual outlet in which the survivor of childhood trauma encapsulates the overwhelming pain and shame of the past, re-enacts salient features of the original events, and copes with the increasingly burdensome demands of selfhood in daily life. Individuals lead conflictual, fragmented lives in which there are many paradoxes. They attempt to escape from pain by harming themselves or others. They want to be wanted but hide their identities behind false identities and ritualized role play. They seek closeness with detached persons who may be thousands of miles away. They seek intense immediate experiences through a medium that ensures depersonalization and objectification.

Eventually, individuals who participate in compulsive sexual behavior experience the "bottoming out" process in which powerlessness and unmanageability confront the illusions of the addictive lifestyle. They can become involved in a recovery process truly dedicated to finding lost parts of oneself by abstaining from compulsive re-enactments and reconstructing the vulnerable self.

TURNING TO OTHERS FOR COMFORT AND SUPPORT

Riso and colleagues[60] suggested that people develop internal working models based on the schema summarized in **Table 1**. Schema are broad pervasive themes comprised of memories, bodily sensations, emotions, and cognitions regarding oneself and one's relationships with others developed during childhood and adolescence and elaborated throughout one's life.

If individuals do not trust others because of attachment trauma and they have the contradictory biologic drive to mate and be sexual, paraphilia solves the problem by allowing them to have sex while distancing themselves with imagery. Masters and Johnson studied sexual arousal patterns of a nonclinical sample and discovered the most common sexual fantasies of both men and women to be (1) sex with strangers and (2) sex with anonymous, faceless partners. Sexual arousal patterns reflect the style of closeness and distance the schema allow. As individuals tolerate greater intimacy, the sexual arousal patterns commonly change. Because changing arousal and fantasy patterns is necessary for comprehensive treatment, changing the schema for trust and safety is essential. In our experience, this begins with clients beginning to trust themselves. One client stated, "I am a liar, cheat, and thief, so I have to assume you are like me." To trust himself, he had to establish greater integrity and not act on self-destructive "dark-side" impulses, which then allowed him to trust others. Sexually out-of-control behavior results in chronic lies to keep the "secrets," which is the germ of self-hatred. Doing what Yolenson and Samenow[61] defined as "opening the channel" and behaving for a period without lying allows the seed for self-empathy to grow.

PARAPHILIA

The terminology for problematic sexual behavior remains confusing. Different terminology is useful, however, in describing a common symptom that derives from a common developmental trajectory. It suggests that clients with the same symptom actually can be more different than they are similar and can require greatly different interventions.

Paraphilia is the most precise term for a variety of out-of-control sexual behaviors. *Para* means "besides," and *philia* means "love," so the term rightly implies a disorder of love, which is experienced as distressing. It suggests that an individual is aroused by atypical sexual imagery or the existence of a sexual object that "intrudes upon or displaces" more common arousal patterns, such as an attractive age mate for which one could hypothetically develop affection. An individual with a leather fetish, for example, finds that leather becomes necessary and distressing because it is requisite for sexual arousal, whereas a desirable partner alone insufficient. Other critical components of paraphilias typically include an element of illicitness;[62] the individual requires secretive behavior, such as paying for rooms in "porn houses," in which strangers perform sexual acts, or engaging in anonymous sex acts in public restrooms, as described in Humphreys'[63] treatise on the "Tea Room Trade." In this manner, the possibility of "being caught" is at once alluring and at the same time provides "evidence" of deserving punishment for being "bad," which often mirrors destructive childhood sexual development in which pleasurable sexual feelings were overpaired with guilt, stigma, or punishment.[55]

Homosexual "tricking," for example, involves multiple sequential partners and is energized by the illicitness and the excitement of "someone" desiring or wanting them. It is a peculiar feature of such acts that the individuals are often so numb or dissociated that the partners chosen are neither attractive nor even sexually arousing to them. Rather it is the "being desired" that is critical. In extreme cases of this behavior within the gay community, the "trick" may even have open HIV sores but sex still takes place, as if the individual is playing Russian roulette with life and death.

Most recently, under the heading of paraphilia, individuals report preoccupation with Internet pornography. This behavior is less "intrusive" in the obsessive imagery sense but still is problematic because it displaces activity with a partner, most commonly their spouse. If such activity involves illegal behavior, the term "sex offender" is used. Some individuals report comorbid depressive and anxiety symptoms that are temporarily ameliorated by the behavior, so the symptom becomes entrenched as a form of affect regulation. Such cases remind the clinician of alcohol or drug addiction because increasingly more activity is needed to satisfy—similar to feelings of withdrawal and tolerance. Individuals often escape into a pleasurable activity temporarily but then recognize that the behavior absorbs increasing dimensions of their life, threatens relationships and employment, and generates hatred. Serotonin reuptake inhibitors often can control such behavior (see the article by Codispoti elsewhere in this issue).

In select cases, the activity looks more like an obsessive-compulsive spectrum disorder characterized by repetitive, driven behaviors that lie along an axis with compulsivity (risk avoidance) and impulsivity (risk and pleasure seeking). The difference between the spectrum disorders lies in the motivation for the repetitive behavior. Disorders at the compulsive end of the spectrum are motivated by harm avoidance and a desire to decrease anxiety. Individuals at the impulsive end are motivated by impulsiveness and a desire to maximize pleasure.[64] The key feature in the labeling of obsessive-compulsive spectrum disorders is that medications such as monoxidase inhibitors can produce almost immediate cessation of the activity, similar to their effect on a hand-washing compulsion.

With paraphilic activity, some clients avoid intimacy because loved ones (the parents) were often sources of danger. Close relationships were necessary but distressing—and still are. For others, sexual acting out is a selfish pursuit of using others, hurting the people they purport to love most, and hurting those they are attracted to. Essentially this manifestation of intimacy is a form of "moving against."[65] Stoller[66] termed such behavior "perversion," indicating the motive was rage and hostility. Such rage is the result of early attachment deficits and childhood abuse and neglect. In such cases, trauma-based psychotherapies are most effective in neutralizing rage and shame. Similar to eating disorders, symptoms such as hypersexual behavior are a complex manifestation of many divergent pathways, the common features being (1) intrusive imagery, (2) displacing partner bonding, (3) a pattern of moving toward, away, or against in bonding, (4) development of the symptom as a form of affect regulation, (5) using the symptom to relieve or combat anxiety or depressive disorder, (6) addictive symptoms characterized by tolerance, withdrawal, habit formation, and interference with work, family life, partner choice, and intimacy, and (7) whether the behavior is illegal.

VANDALIZED LOVE MAP

The unique aspect of sexuality in comparison to other natural functions is the cementing of arousal patterns and fantasy during adolescence. John Money[67] defined these arousal patterns more broadly as love maps: "a personalized developmental representation or template in the mind or in the brain that depicts the idealized lover and the idealized program of sexuoerotic activity with the lover as projected in imagery and idealization or actually engaged in with that lover." Money pioneered the study of structural and developmental contributions to the affectional systems. Like Bowlby, Money believed that actual biographic events related to attachment and trauma influence the development of a love map that can become "vandalized." Too much punishment associated with genital sexuality and out-of-control premature sexualization in the household constitute two examples.

The developing love map encompasses proceptive events, such as the range of partner characteristics that sexually arouse the body to respond to touch or genitals to respond to various stimuli and the sense of self as attractive, which obviously influences the perception of others as pleasurable. Some theorists assert that deviation in the development of proceptive love maps become "delayed," "fixated," or "regressed," whereas others suggest that deviant development continues but along a different, distinct, or complex route.[68] The love map of child molesters has been labeled "fixated" by some theorists and viewed as requiring unblocking; alternatively, it may have differentiated along a distinct pathway.[69] Within a developmental psychopathology frame, such deviation can be understood only by looking at normal development (ie, secure attachment modulated impulse control, adaptive temperament, entry into peer group, and dating). Pathology reflects repeated failure of adaptation with respect to these issues. Change or resilience is also possible at many points. Puberty activates the "love map" established throughout childhood. Abel and colleagues[70] evaluated 411 adult sex offenders in an outpatient clinic. Of this sample, 58% reported that their deviant sexual arousal began before age 18. Other studies of juvenile offenders found that age of onset ranged from 13 to 15 years[71] and included a wide variety of paraphilias, including molestation, voyeurism, exhibitionism, obscene phone calls, and transvestism, some of which began as early as 10 years of age.

PSYCHODYNAMICS

Stoller[66] considered sexually compulsive behavior a "perversion," that is "the erotic form of hatred that serves the function of revenge." He stated that the perversion serves a survival role by converting childhood trauma to triumph. The person seeks sexual release without genuinely caring about the sexual partner and with little empathetic connection to self or other. The goal is to fulfill an appetite regardless of other. Sometimes pleasure is even derived from degrading the other or self. In such cases, suppressed affect is misdirected at oneself, one's body, one's genitals, one's gender, or one's partner.

The "triumph over tragedy" is the result of repetition with the erotic theme of control. In this way, sexually acting out is much like another form of being in charge of one's pain, self-cutting, a reasonable adaptation to the double-bind polarizations of needing caretaking but fearing dependency, or needing sexual release while being terrified of closeness. It allows for intimacy without connection as a survival solution to feared annihilation. For example, one client discussed a shameful sexual liaison that resulted in his being urinated on consensually. The feelings of degradation were re-experienced under hypnosis and then used to bridge him to an age-regressed state. He began to relive an incident that occurred when he was a child and the school bully beat him up and urinated on him. At around the same age, he was used by his older brother as a sexual outlet, and peers were teasing him in other cruel ways. His brother confirmed the memories. By working with the intense affect and reliving the shame of the encounter, the client's sexual arousal for urophilia diminished. Most cases of sexually compulsive ego states begin in adolescence,[72] and often it is the adolescent self that holds the deviant arousal. From a developmental perspective, if bonding and sexuality are introduced to a child with contradictory affect, cognition, and behavior, it is likely to remain intertwined in the "hard drive" of the brain.

SEXUALIZED CHILDREN

Two changes are occurring in contemporary families. One is the increasing overindulgence of children by buying them products to compensate for parental neglect and absences. Frequently, overindulgence is accompanied by overcontrol, in which a parent is also enmeshed with the child and has highly perfectionistic performance concerns for achievement. It is as if the child is "fed but not nourished." Such families are often chaotic and the attachments are disorganized. The cost of surviving in such families often involves giving up development of an autonomous self; rarely does their self-sufficient parenting allow natural maturation. These children are needy and develop strong dependency in relationships, wanting to merge while simultaneously feeling it necessary to run away out of fear of rejection and loss of control. Such individuals have a poor sense of self or identity. They continually seek attachments to finish the self—two halves making a whole—but the relationships are conflicted. Sexuality seems premature in such relationships and can be experienced as traumatic because these individuals are immature for their age. It is not uncommon in the treatment of exhibitionists or voyeurs to find that their primary relationship even in childhood was with their mother and they still live at home. They feel like this relationship is necessary but distressing.

The second change is the premature sexualization of children through exposure to eroticism by family, media, and role expectations. Children are also reaching puberty earlier, and John Fowles wrote, "It is as if a ship is sent to sea without a rudder." Kids are genitally and socially eroticized without sufficient guidance and launching for attachments (ie, "love education"). The result is that children can be exposed to sexuality and look okay on the outside but be traumatized internally by premature sexual and love experiences.

In such cases, vulnerable children may be genitally activated but make poor decisions that will change their lives. They may sell themselves for "tricks" in the homosexual community, seek out contact with neighborhood pedophiles, molest siblings or peers, or flirt on the Internet. Such individuals often confuse the need for affection with sexual arousal. This tendency is exacerbated by the media's frequent and sensationalized use of sexuality to get the attention of children and adolescents without the ameliorating influence of parental guidance. Sibling or peer group pressure further encourages "sexualized children," who experiment with sexual behaviors before they are emotionally ready.

ADDICTIVE CYCLES

Early attachment disorganization is experienced by adults as numbness, constriction, and feeling object-like, mechanical, and empty—all of which propel them to seek relief, escape, and connection. Such individuals were labeled "bypassers" by Masters and Johnson[73] because they became sexually aroused reflexively without much attraction or affection for their partners. Typically, such individuals feel internal polarities of dependency—needs that feel insatiable because of childhood neglect and are often experienced as terrifying. They exert "control" that results in periods of hyposexuality because of a fear of intimacy. Eventually the natural desire to escape their loneliness and bond takes over and they enter a release phase of being out of control and hypersexual. It is common to see such individuals cycle, much like the anorexic-binge type, from what appears as "sexual anorexia" to sexual out of control (bingeing)—overcontrol/out-of-control cycles. In some ways, sex is objectifying and depersonalizing and nonintimate, so after the release of orgasm, emptiness quickly follows, which requires another "hit." This cycle can seem "addictive" because individuals quickly cycle from the high (some illusion of connection or escape from emptiness) to the deep loss of profound aloneness.

This pattern is most common within the gay community through anonymous sex scenes or bath houses in which individuals have sex multiple times in an evening. However, it has become increasingly common with cybersex addictions in which individuals masturbate to their computer screens. In a large sample, 96% of men and women reported feeling addicted to Internet sex and spent more than 11 hours a week on sexual online activity.[70,74,75] In 1999, there were 19,542,710 visitors a month on the top five pay pornography sites; 70% of that number visited on weekdays between 9AM and 5PM. Currently, approximately 40 million Americans admit to regularly visiting pornography Web sites.

REFERENCES

1. Money J. Lovemaps: clinical concepts of sexual erotic health and pathology, paraphilia, and gender transposition of childhood, adolescence, and maturity. New York: Irvington; 1986.
2. Marshall WL. The role of attachment, intimacy, and loneliness in the etiology and maintance of sexual offenders. Sex Marital Ther 1993;8:109–21.
3. Marshall WL, Serran GA, Costins FA. Childhood attachment, sexual abuse, and their relationship to adult coping in child molesters. Sex Abuse 2000;12:17–26.
4. Marshall WL. Intimacy, loneliness, and sexual offenders. Behavioral Resolution Therapy 1989;27:491–503.
5. Laws DR, Marshall WL. A conditioning theory of the etiology and maintenance of deviant sexual preference and behavior. In: Marshall WL, Laws DR, Barabree HE, editors. Handbook of sexual assault: issues, theories and treatment of the offender. New York: Putnam; 1990. p. 209–30.
6. Marshall W, Barbaeu H. Sexual violence: clinical approaches to violence. New York: Wiley; 1989. p. 205–45.
7. Cloninger CR. Brain networks underlying personality development. In: Carroll BJ, Barrett JE, editors. Psychopathology and the brain. New York: Raven Press; 1991. p. 183–208.
8. Cucchetti D, Cohen DJ. Developmental psychopathology: theory and method. New York: John Wiley & Sons; 1995.
9. Jensen P, Hoagwood K. The book of names: PSM-IV in context. Developmental Psychopathology 1997;9:231–6.
10. Schwartz M, Galperin L, Schwartz R. Systemically based individual psychotherapy for complex traumatic stress disorders. Complex traumatic stress disorders: an evidence-based clinician's guide. New York: Guilford Press; 2007.
11. Abel N, Roulean J. The nature and extent of sexual assault. In: Marshall W, Lewis R, editors. Handbook of sexual assault. New York: Plenery; 1990. p. 150–65.

12. Knight RA, Prentreg RA. Classifying sexual offenders. In: Marshall WL, Laws DR, Barbaree HE, editors. Handbook of sexual assault. New York: Plenum; 1990. p. 20–35.

13. Cloninger R, Bayon C, Svrakic D. Measurement of temperament and character in mood disorders: a model of fundamental states as personality types. J Affect Disord 1998;51(1):21–32.

14. Caspi A, Lynam D, Moffitt TE, et al. Unraveling girls' delinquency: biological, dispositional, and contextual contributions to adolescent misbehavior. Dev Psychol 1993;29(1):19–30.

15. Cloninger CR. A systemic method for clinical description and classification of personality traits. Arch Gen Psychiatry 1987;44(6):573–83.

16. Hammock GS, Richardson DR. Perceptions of rape: the influence of closeness of relationship, intoxication, and sex of participant. Violence Vict 1997;12: 237–46.

17. Malamethy M, Sockloskie R. Characteristics of aggressors against women and clinical psychology. Journal of Consulting and Clinical Psychology 1991;59(5): 670–81.

18. Rapaport K, Burkhard B. Personality and attitudinal characteristics of sexually coercive collage males. J Abnorm Psychol 1987;93(2):216–21.

19. Freund K. Assessment of pedophilia. In: Cooke M, Howell K, editors. Adult interest in children. London: Academic Press; 1981. p. 139–71.

20. Marshall W. A revised approach to the treatment of men who sexually assault females. In: Hall G, Hirschman R, Graham J, editors. Sexual aggression issues in etiology assessment and treatment; 1993. p. 143–65.

21. Fehrenbach P, Monastersky C. Characteristics of female adolescent sexual offenders. Am J Orthopsychiatry 1988;58(1):148–51.

22. Schwartz MF, Mark F, Galperin LD, et al. Dissociation and treatment of compulsive reenactment of trauma: sexual compulsivity. In: Hunter M, editor. Adult survivors of sexual abuse: treatment innovation. Thousand Oaks (CA): Sage Publications, Inc; 1995. p. 42–55.

23. Schore A. Affect regulation and the origin of self: the neurobiology of emotional development. Hillsdale (UK): Lawrence Erlbaum Associates, Inc.; 1994.

24. Maclean P, Kral V. A triune concept of the brain and behavior. In: Boag T, editor. Toronto (ON): Toronto University; 1973.

25. Fosha D. Dyadic regulations and experiential work with emotion and relatedness in trauma and disorganized attachment. In: Solomon M, Siegel D, editors. Healing trauma: attachment, mind, body, and brain. New York: W.W. Norton & Company, Inc.; 2003. p. 221–81.

26. Bowlby J. Attachment and loss, separation. New York: Basic Books; 1973.

27. Kobak R, Hazan C. Attachment in marriage: effects of security and accuracy of working models. J Pers Soc Psychol 1991;60:861–9.

28. Stroufe A. Emotional Development: the organization of emotional life in the early years. Cambridge (UK): Cambridge University Press; 1995.

29. Greenspan S. Developmentally based psychotherapy. Madison (CT): International University Press; 1997.

30. Sroufe LA. Infant–caregiver attachment and patterns of adaptation in preschool: the roots of maladaptation and competence. In: Palmetta M, editor. Development and policy concerning children with special needs: the Minnesota symposia on child psychology. New York: Lawrence Erlbaum; 1981. p. 41–84.

31. Main M, Solomon J. Procedures for identifying infants as disorganized/disoriented during the Ainsworth strange situation. In: Greenberg M, Cucchette D,

editors. Attachment during the preschool years. Chicago: University of Chicago Press; 1990. p. 121–60.

32. Ogawa N, Stroufe A, Weinfield E, et al. Development and fragmented self: longitudinal study of dissociative symptomatology in a nonclinical sample. Dev Psychopathol 1997;9:855–79.

33. Marshall WL, Laws DR. A brief history of behavioral and cognitive approaches to sexual offender treatment. Sex Abuse 2003;15:93–120.

34. Mahler MS. The psychological birth of the human infant: symbiotic and individualization. New York: Basic Books; 1975.

35. Sroufe LA, Waters E. Attachment as an organizational construct. Child Dev 1979; 48:1189–99.

36. Epstein S. Cognitive-experimental self therapy. In: Pervin LA, editor. Handbook of personality. New York: Guilford Press; 1997. p. 165–1929.

37. Marshall W, Eccles A. The assessment and treatment of adolescent sex offenders: pavlovian conditioning processes in adolescent sex offenders. In: Marshall WL, Laws DR, Barbaree HE, editors. Handbook of sexual assault: issues, theories, and treatment of the offender. New York: Plenum Press; 1993. p. 95–102.

38. Prentky RA, Knight R, Sims-Knight JE, et al. Development antecedents to sexual neglect and violent sex offender aggression. Development and Psychopathology 1989;1(2):153–69.

39. Fonagy P, Gergeloy G, Jurist E, et al. Affect regulation, metalization and the development of self. New York: Other Press; 2002.

40. Sroufe L. An organizational perspective on the self. In: Cicchetti D, Beeghly M, editors. The self in transition: infancy to childhood. Chicago: University of Chicago Press; 1990. p. 281–307.

41. Putnam FW. Dissociation in children and adolescents. New York: Guilford Press; 1997.

42. Sroufe LA. Emotional development: the organization of emotional life in the early years. Cambridge (UK): Cambridge University Press; 1996.

43. Herman J. Sex offenders: a feminist perspective. In: Marshall WL, Laws DR, Barbaree HE, editors. Handbook of sexual assault: issues, theories, and treatment of the offender. New York: Plenum Press; 1990. p. 177–93.

44. Miller A. Banished knowledge. New York: Doubleday; 1990.

45. Putnam FW. Diagnosis and treatment of multiple personality disorder. New York: Guilford Press; 1989.

46. Yehuda R, McFarland A. Psychobiology of post traumatic stress. New York: Academy of Science; 1998.

47. Terr LC. Childhood traumas: an outline and overview. Am J Psychiatry 1991;148: 10–20.

48. Van der Kolk BA. The compulsion to repeat the trauma, reenactment, revictimization and masoclusion. Psychiatr Clin North Am 1989;12:389–411.

49. Wallin D. Attachment in psychotherapy. New York: Guilford; 2007.

50. Horowitz M. Stress-response syndromes: a review of posttraumatic and adjustment disorders. American Psychiatric Association 1986;37:241–9.

51. Schwartz MF. Reenactment related to bonding and hypersexuality. Sexual Addiction and Compulsivity 1996;3:195–212.

52. Van der Kolk BA. The body keeps the score. In: Van der Kolk BA, editor. Traumatic stress: the effects of overwhelming experience over mind, body and society. New York: Guilford Press; 1996. p. 214–41.

53. Schwartz M. Victim to victimizer. Professional Counselor 1991;1:44–50.

54. Horowitz MJ. Stress response syndromes: personality styles and interventions. Lanham (MD): Jason Aronson Publishing, Inc.; 1976.

55. Hindman. Just before dawn: trauma assessment and sexual victimization. Lincoln City (OR): Alexandria Associates; 1989.

56. Van der Kolk B, McFarlane A, Weisaeth L. Traumatic stress. New York: Guilford Press; 1996.

57. Schwartz MF, Becklin R. Sexually evoked aggression of aggression–induced sex in the rhesus monkey. Cornell J Soc Relat 1975;7:117–31.

58. Frederick W, Luecke W. Young school age sexually aggressive children. Prof Psychol 1988;19:155–64.

59. Watkins JG, Watkins HH. Ego states: theory and therapy. New York: WW Norton; 1997.

60. Riso LP, du Toit PL, Stein DJ, Young JE, editors. Cognitive schemas and core beliefs in psychological problems: a scientist-practitioner guide. Washington (DC): American Psychological Association; 2007.

61. Yolenson S, Samenow J. The criminal personality. New York: Jason Aronson; 1977.

62. Schwartz MF, Southern S. Compulsive cybersex: the new tea room. In: Cooper A, editor. Cybersex: the dark side of the force. New York: Routledge; 2000. p. 127–44.

63. Humphreys L. The tearoom trade. Chicago: Aldine Press; 1970.

64. Van der Kolk B. Dissociation, somatization and affect dyregulation. Journal of Psychiatry 1996;153:83–93.

65. Horney K. Our inner conflicts, a constructive theory of neurosis. New York: W. W. Norton & Company, Inc.; 1945.

66. Stoller R. Perversion. London: Karnac Books; 1986.

67. Money J. Lovemaps: clinical concepts of sexual/erotic health and pathology, paraphilia, and gender transposition, childhood, adolescence, and maturity. New York: Irving Publishers; 1986.

68. Hollander E, Rosen J. Impulsivity. J Psychopharmacol 2000;14:539–44.

69. Groth A, Hobson W, Gary T. The child molester: clinical observations. In: Conte J, Shore D, editors. Social work and child sexual abuse. Binghampton (NY): The Haworth Press; 1982. p. 129–44.

70. Abel G, Mittelman M, Becker J. Of sexual arousal in several paraphilias. Behavioral Res Therapy 1985;19:25–33.

71. Becker JV, Kaplan MS, Kavoussi R. Measuring the effectiveness of treatment for the aggressive adolescent sex offender. Annals of the New York Academy of Sciences 1988;528:215–22.

72. Awad G, Saunder EB. Adolescent child molesters. Child Psychiatry Hum Dev 1989;19:195–206.

73. Masters W, Johnson VE. Human sexual inadequacy. Boston: Little Brown; 1971.

74. Schwartz MF, Masters WH. Integration of trauma-based, cognitive, behavioral, systemic and addiction approaches for treatment of hypersexual pair-bonding disorder. Sexual Addiction and Compulsivity 1994;1:57–76.

75. Cooper A. Sexuality and the Internet. Cyberpsychol Behav 1998;1:181–7.

Classifying Hypersexual Disorders: Compulsive, Impulsive, and Addictive Models

Dan J. Stein, MD, PhD[a,b,*]

KEYWORDS

- Hypersexual disorder • Sexual addiction • Compulsive
- Impulsive

There is a range of variation in sexual activity. People with clinically excessive sexual thoughts or behaviors have been categorized as suffering from a compulsive, impulsive, or addictive sexual disorder. Such terms reflect key theoretical assumptions about the nature of the behavior. Thus, some have described compulsive sexual symptoms and addressed their relationship to obsessive-compulsive disorder[1]. Others have emphasized the role of impulsivity, and the spectrum of impulse control disorders, in conceptualizing such symptoms.[2] Finally, DSM-III-R used the term non-paraphilic sexual addiction,[3] an approach consistent with one that emphasizes the addictive nature of these symptoms, but inconsistent with the decision not to include this term in DSM-IV.

Similar considerations apply to the symptoms of a range of conditions included in the DSM category of impulse control disorders not otherwise classified. These disorders include intermittent explosive disorder, kleptomania, pathological gambling, pyromania, and trichotillomania. Thus, for example, clinically excessive gambling has been described as compulsive, impulsive, or addictive.[4] Similarly, clinically excessive hair-pulling has been characterized as compulsive, impulsive, and addictive.[5] Thus it seems that the phenomenology and psychobiology of these conditions remains incompletely understood, with a range of different nosological terminology and conceptual models still under active consideration by the field.

In this article we consider the nosological implications of advances in understanding the phenomenology and psychobiology of the non-paraphilic sexual addictions and the impulse control disorders not otherwise classified. We argue that each of the compulsive, impulsive, and addictive approaches seems to offer only a partial view of these conditions. We go on to review research suggesting that key components of such conditions include affective dysregulation (A), behavioral addiction (B), and cognitive dyscontrol (C). We then use this research to argue for a revision of the

[a] University of Cape Town, Private Bag X3, Rondebosch 7701, Cape Town, South Africa
[b] Mt. Sinai School of Medicine, 5 East 98th Street, New York, NY 10029, USA
* University of Cape Town, Private Bag X3, Rondebosch 7701, Cape Town, South Africa.
E-mail address: dan.stein@uct.ac.za

Psychiatr Clin N Am 31 (2008) 587–591
doi:10.1016/j.psc.2008.06.007
0193-953X/08/$ – see front matter © 2008 Elsevier Inc. All rights reserved.

nomenclature of these conditions, and to advocate for additional work on their classification and pathogenesis.

COMPULSIVE-IMPULSIVE-ADDICTIVE VIEWS OF SEXUAL SYMPTOMS

Obsessive-compulsive disorder (OCD) is perhaps the paradigmatic compulsive disorder. It is characterized by obsessions (intrusive thoughts, images, or impulses), and compulsions (repetitive thoughts or actions that act to neutralize the obsessions). Typically obsessions increase anxiety, while compulsions decrease anxiety. Compulsive sexual symptoms are also characterized by repetitiveness, with an increase in tension before the behavior, and a sense of release at the time of their execution. Although OCD behavior is typically characterized by dysphoria, and sexual behavior by gratification, there are inter-individual differences (some OCD patients describe a "just right" feeling, and many patients with compulsive sexual symptoms describe guilt and regret).[6]

Impulsive personality disorders are perhaps the paradigmatic impulsive condition. They are characterized by various kinds of impulsivity, including hyperresponsiveness to stress, inability to delay gratification, and impulsive decision making. Similarly, patients with clinically excessive sexual thoughts and behaviors may have an increase in symptoms in response to stress, may demonstrate an inability to delay sexual gratification, and may have impulsive decision making in a range of situations including those involving sex. As noted below, a range of other impulse control disorders may also demonstrate these elements; the temper outbursts of intermittent explosive disorder, for example, may be exacerbated at times of stress, may be associated with inability to delay gratification, and may reflect poor executive control.[7]

Substance dependence is the paradigmatic addictive disorder. Patients with substance dependence are preoccupied with obtaining more substances, attempt to consume more and more of a particular substance to get the same "high," and demonstrate withdrawal symptoms after abrupt discontinuation of their symptoms. Similarly, patients with clinically excessive sexual thoughts or behaviors are preoccupied with their concerns, may demonstrate an escalating pattern of symptoms, and experience dysphoria when they attempt to discontinue their behaviors.[8] It is not surprising, then, that a number of authors have conceptualized such symptoms as addictive in nature, and that 12-step programs based on models for addressing substance use disorders have been proposed for their treatment.

There are important problems with each of these conceptual approaches to clinically excessive sexual thoughts or behaviors. First, there are subtle but important distinctions between these symptoms and those seen in the paradigmatic compulsive, impulsive, and addictive disorders. The typical behaviors of OCD do not involve reward (unlike sexual behavior), the impulsive personality may be unable to plan carefully to achieve goals (such as sexual encounters), and substance use disorders crucially involve a substance (rather than simply a rewarding behavior like sex). Second, there may be important distinctions in the psychobiology of these disorders; for example, whereas OCD is mediated by cortico-striatal-thalamic circuitry, the role of these pathways in excessive sexual symptoms is less clear. Third, the standard treatments for some of these conditions (eg, exposure and response prevention in OCD) may differ from those thought to be effective in excessive sexual symptoms.

AN A-B-C MODEL OF IMPULSE CONTROL DISORDERS

We have proposed that key components of impulse control disorders, such as trichotillomania, include affective dysregulation (A), behavioral addiction (B), and cognitive dyscontrol (C).[7] We briefly describe each of these components next.

Affective dysregulation appears to be an important trigger of many of the symptoms of the impulse control disorders not otherwise specified. Thus patients with trichotillomania note that hair-pulling is often triggered by negative affects. Similar associations are described in other impulse control disorders (ICDs) such as pathological gambling. There is growing interest in the psychobiology of stress-induced impulsivity, and it can be hypothesized that amygdala activation may play a particularly important role. It is possible that selective serotonin reuptake inhibitors are effective in some ICDs precisely because they act on such circuitry, and help to modulate affect dysregulation.

Many of the ICDs can be described as "behavioral addictions" insofar as patients demonstrate a preoccupation with their symptoms, there may a gradual increase in symptom severity consistent with tolerance, and there is considerable dysphoria should symptoms be discontinued. It is notable that ventral striatal circuitry, and the nucleus accumbens in particular, may play an important role in mediating not only substance use disorders, but also a range of symptoms seen in impulse control disorders. It is possible that dopamine blockers are effective in some ICDs precisely because they act on such circuitry, and help to modulate behavioral addiction.

Many of the ICDs may be characterized by cognitive dyscontrol. At a clinical level, patients seem unable to fully cognitively and affectively process the medium and long-term consequences of acting on their impulses. At a neuropsychological level, there is often evidence of impaired executive control on systematic testing. At a biological level, there may be evidence of decreased prefrontal activation in patients with such cognitive dyscontrol, supporting the evidence that symptoms result from impaired executive control. It is possible that anticonvulsant (or neurostabilizer) medications are effective in some ICDs precisely because they act on such circuitry, and help to reduce cognitive dyscontrol.

An A-B-C model of the ICDs suggests that instead of taking a single theoretical approach to the classification and understanding of these conditions (whether compulsive, impulsive, or addictive), it may instead be useful to explore the different phenomenological and psychobiological components that underpin these conditions. First, instead of reducing symptoms to a single kind of category, it would allow an exploration of a range of phenomena seen in these disorders, as well as their comorbidity. Second, instead of explaining symptoms using only a particular set of neurocircuitry and related neurochemistry, it would allow various pathways to be explored. Third, by outlining a range of different target phenomena, it would encourage the exploration of a number of different therapeutic interventions for these conditions.

AN A-B-C MODEL OF HYPERSEXUAL DISORDER

These considerations suggest that an A-B-C model of clinically excessive sexual thoughts and behaviors may be useful and such symptoms should be described in a theoretically neutral way. The term "hypersexual disorder," for example, does not rely on the compulsive, impulsive, or addictive models, and so allows each of these approaches to be explored in relation to sexual symptoms. In the absence of clear agreement on how best to conceptualize the phenomenology and psychobiology of hypersexual disorder, a theoretically neutral term may be particularly useful in encouraging a range of approaches in both clinical settings and in the research laboratory.[9]

Furthermore, various data suggest that affective dysregulation may play an important role in hypersexual disorder. First, symptoms may be triggered or exacerbated during times of increased stress and affective arousal. Second, many patients with hypersexual disorder have comorbid mood and anxiety disorders.[1] Third, the selective serotonin reuptake inhibitors (SSRIs) that are useful in modulating affect, and in treating a range of mood and anxiety disorders, appear to also be useful in decreasing symptoms of hypersexual disorder—even in patients with comorbidity of these disorders.[10,11]

A number of arguments can also be put forward to support the hypothesis that behavioral addiction is relevant to hypersexual disorder. In particular, as described earlier, patients with hypersexual disorder may be preoccupied with their sexual desires, may demonstrate an escalating pattern of acting on such desires, and may exhibit significant dysphoria when they attempt to cut back on their behaviors. Although the relative paucity of psychobiological research on hypersexual disorder makes it difficult to conclude that neurocircuitry relevant to behavioral addiction plays a role in mediating this condition, it is notable that pro-dopaminergic drugs may increase sexual behavior.

Finally, there is at least some evidence that cognitive dyscontrol may play a role in hypersexual disorder. Although there is again a paucity of systematic psychobiological research on this condition, there is evidence that executive functions are impaired in patients with paraphilias. Certainly, there is anecdotal evidence that patients with hypersexual disorder are unable to process optimally the consequences of their actions. Although additional research is clearly needed, such considerations raise the question of whether anticonvulsant or neuromodulator agents that act on glutamatergic and GABAergic circuitry, and may be useful in a range of impulse control disorders, may also be useful in hypersexual disorder.

SUMMARY

In closing, we argue for two conclusions. First, there are advantages to using theoretically neutral terms (such as hypersexual disorder) that go beyond the compulsive-impulsive-addictive distinctions.[9] Although the notion of theory-neutral observation cannot be defended, it is important not to rely on any particular theoretical framework before all the evidence is in. Our current nosology employs a range of contradictory terms and frameworks (eg, *impulse* control disorder, *compulsive* gambling and buying, trichotillo*mania,* and klepto*mania*). In keeping with the approach taken in other DSM categories, it may be useful to find a more theory-neutral term that can cut across these conditions.

Second, any conclusions drawn here about the nosology of hypersexual disorder must be tempered by the relative lack of rigorous psychobiological and systematic treatment data. A better understanding of the psychobiology of hypersexual disorder might provide greater confidence in one or the other theoretical model. The A-B-C model proposed here is tentative at best, given the relative absence of supporting data. Further, a richer assessment and treatment literature would allow clearer conclusions about the clinical utility of different nosological approaches. We emphasize the need for much additional work to characterize the phenomenology and psychobiology of hypersexual disorder and other conditions characterized by affective dysregulation, behavioral addiction, and cognitive dyscontrol, in the hope that such research would ultimately lead to improved assessment and management.

ACKNOWLEDGMENTS

Dr. Stein is supported by the Medical Research Council of South Africa.

REFERENCES

1. Black DW, Kehrberg LL, Flumerfelt DL, et al. Characteristics of 36 subjects reporting compulsive sexual behavior. Am J Psychiatry 1997;154:243–9.

2. McElroy SL, Phillips KA, Keck PE Jr. Obsessive compulsive spectrum disorder. J Clin Psychiatry 1994;55(Suppl):33–51.
3. American Psychiatric Association. Diagnostic and statistical manual of mental disorders. 3rd (revised) edition. Washington, DC: American Psychiatric Association; 1987.
4. Grant JE, Potenza MN. Pathological gambling: a clinical guide to treatment. Washington, DC: APPI; 2004.
5. Stein DJ, Mullen L, Islam MN, et al. Compulsive and impulsive symptomatology in trichotillomania. Psychopathology 1995;28:208–13.
6. Lochner C, Stein DJ. Does work on obsessive-compulsive spectrum disorders contribute to understanding the heterogeneity of obsessive-compulsive disorder? Prog Neuropsychopharmacol Biol Psychiatry 2006;30:353–61.
7. Stein DJ, Chamberlain SR, Fineberg N. An A-B-C model of habit disorders: hair-pulling, skin-picking, and other stereotypic conditions. CNS Spectr 2006;11: 824–7.
8. Goodman A. Sexual addiction: An integrated approach. Madison, CT: International Universities Press; 1998.
9. Stein DJ, Black DW, Shapira NA, et al. Hypersexual disorder and preoccupation with Internet pornography. Am J Psychiatry 2001;158:1590–4.
10. Stein DJ, Hollander E, Anthony D, et al. Serotonergic medications for sexual obsessions, sexual addictions, and paraphilias. J Clin Psychiatry 1992;53:267–71.
11. Kafka M: Psychopharmacological treatments for nonparaphilic compulsive sexual behaviors. CNS Spectr 2000;5:49–59.

Sexual Behavior that is "Out of Control": a Theoretical Conceptual Approach

John Bancroft, MD[a,b]

KEYWORDS

- Sexual behavior • Negative mood • Sexual arousal
- Self-regulation • Out of control

Sexual behavior that is, in some sense, "out-of-control" can result in a variety of problems. Damage to relationships, interference with work, loss of time and money, and negative impact on self-esteem are common examples. Sexual behavior that breaks the law, known as a sexual offense, can also be deemed out of control, but that category of sexual behavior is excluded from discussion in this article.

In the past, a variety of labels have been used to describe out-of-control sexual behavior, such as nymphomania, satyriasis, and hypersexuality.[1] More recently two concepts have prevailed: "compulsive sexual behavior" and "sexual addiction." Barth and Kinder[2] argued for the use of "impulse control disorder" as a description. Unlike the "compulsivity" and "addiction" labels, this would be consistent with DSM criteria, but beyond inferring a problem of self-control, it has little explanatory value. The literature on "sexual compulsivity" and "sexual addiction" has been preoccupied with definitions, particularly as pertain to DSM-IV criteria, rather than working to explain how and why, in such cases, sexual behavior becomes problematic. Statements are often made about likely mechanisms, eg, anxiety reduction or mood regulation, but these are based more on clinical impression than reported data. This has led Gold and Heffner[3] to title their review paper "Sexual Addictions: Many Conceptions, Minimal Data."

Explaining how and why sexual behavior gets out of control is fundamentally important to the advancement of effective treatments. In this article, some explanatory theoretical concepts are discussed, and relevant data (although limited) are considered. At this point, however, we are at the stage of formulating testable hypotheses, and data remains minimal.

Two types of sexual behavior are most likely to become out of control: masturbation, probably the most common, and various kinds of behavioral interactions with

[a] The Kinsey Institute for Research in Sex, Gender and Reproduction, Indiana University, Bloomington, IN, USA
[b] Barnhurst, 4 Blenheim Road, Horspath, Oxfordshire, OX33 1RY, UK
E-mail address: jbancrof@indiana.edu

Psychiatr Clin N Am 31 (2008) 593–601
doi:10.1016/j.psc.2008.06.009
0193-953X/08/$ – see front matter © 2008 Elsevier Inc. All rights reserved.

others. A new and exceedingly important development is the sexual use of the Internet. A large and growing number of both men and women use the Internet for sexual purposes. Men are more likely to access sexually explicit material online; women use it more for interactions or cybersex.[4] Most persons are able to use the Internet for sexual purposes without it becoming a problem, or out of control. But for those affected, out of control Internet sex is the fastest growing aspect of this problem area. The Internet is unique in that it allows and even encourages a blending of the "masturbatory" and "interactive" patterns referred to above. Men, in particular, use the Internet as an almost limitless extension of their out of control masturbatory behavior. For others, social interaction via chat rooms and other online networking remains important although masturbation is likely to be the principal pattern of sexual release. Internet interactions allow considerable modifications and variations in how one presents one's self (the construction of a false self), and how one interacts, yet little is currently known about how this contributes to the undermining of self-control. A collection of essays on the topic has been edited by Cooper.[5]

We also have limited data on what makes a person vulnerable to loss of sexual control. Raviv[6] found that 32 self-identified "sex addicts" had higher mean scores on SCL-90-R scales for anxiety, depression, obsessive-compulsiveness, and interpersonal sensitivity, than 38 controls. In an uncontrolled study of 37 subjects with self-defined out-of-control sexual behavior, Black and colleagues,[7] found a high prevalence of comorbidity with psychiatric conditions, most notably lifetime histories of substance use disorders (64%), anxiety disorders (50%), and mood disorders (39%). Quadland[8] compared 30 gay men presenting for treatment for compulsive sexual behavior with an age-matched group of 24 gay men who were presenting for treatment for nonsexual problems. He found differences in their patterns of sexual behavior (eg, number of sexual partners and duration of sexual relationships), but no group differences in mood or personality disorder.

There is increasing evidence that out-of-control sexual behavior can be reduced by mood-elevating drugs such as selective serotonin reuptake inhibitors (SSRIs),[9-11] supporting the idea that the problem is mood related, at least in a proportion of cases. However, we do not yet know to what extent such pharmacological benefits result from improvement in mood, inhibition of sexual response, or both. Given the high prevalence of sexual side effects with such drugs,[12] serotonergic inhibition of sexual response is likely to be relevant.

Recent research at the Kinsey Institute has focused on the role of sexual excitation and inhibition and the impact of negative mood on sexual risk-taking as well as sexual dysfunctions.[13,14] The Institute conducted a small study of 29 male and 2 female self-defined sex addicts[15] who were interviewed and completed questionnaires. Their questionnaire data were compared with a large age-matched control group. This study provided the starting point for postulating a range of possible causal mechanisms that lead to sexual behavior becoming out of control. These will be briefly reviewed here, with illustrations from that study, hereafter referred to as our sex addicts study. The mechanisms listed include (1) impact of negative mood; (2) impaired inhibition of sexual arousal; (3) impaired self-regulation; (4) out-of-control sexual behavior as a sexual addiction; and (5) out-of-control sexual behavior as an obsessive-compulsive disorder.

IMPACT OF NEGATIVE MOOD

For most people, negative mood in terms of both depression and anxiety is associated with reduced sexual interest and/or response. A minority of individuals, however, report the paradoxical tendency for sexual feelings to be increased during negative mood states. Until recently, most of the relevant evidence came from studies of clinical affective disorders (reviewed in Bancroft and colleagues).[16] The impact of depression and anxiety in nonclinical groups has now been explored using a simple instrument, the Mood and Sexuality Questionnaire (MSQ).[16] Covering both depression and anxiety, and sexual interest and sexual response, the MSQ uses four questions: "When you have felt depressed (or anxious/stressed) what typically happens to your sexual interest" (or response)? A bipolar 1 to 9 scale is used, with 5 indicating no change, and 9 a marked increase. In studies of heterosexual men,[16] gay men,[17] and heterosexual women,[18] around 10% of men and women reported increased sexual interest when depressed, and around 20% when anxious or stressed. Qualitative data indicated a more complex relationship between depression and sexuality, and a comparatively simple relationship with anxiety, most commonly expressed by masturbation.[16,17] These relationships will be considered further below.

What is the relevance of this paradoxical mood-sexuality relationship to out-of-control sexual behavior? In our sex addicts study,[15] 27 subjects (87%) stated that their sexual acting out was predictably affected by their mood. Seventeen subjects reported being more likely to sexually act out when depressed, and 19 when anxious or stressed. Eleven subjects (nine men and two women) reported an increase in "acting out" in states of both depression and anxiety. Two men said that they were less likely to act out when depressed; no one said this in relation to anxiety. As a group, their scores on the MSQ were significantly higher than those of the controls ($P < .001$), indicating their greater likelihood of being sexually responsive in negative mood states. These sex addicts also scored significantly higher on a trait measure of proneness to depression.

An association between negative mood and out-of-control sexual behavior therefore appears to be highly relevant. However, based on qualitative data from our larger studies,[16,17] this is not simply "using sex as a mood regulator." A number of mediating mechanisms may be involved. Three patterns can be considered:

1. Persons who retain sexual interest or responsiveness in states of depression might be pursuing sexual contact with another person to satisfy depression-related emotional needs, such as making personal contact through sex, feeling validated by another person, and enhancing one's self-esteem by feeling desired by another person. These are direct examples of mood regulation.
2. Sexual stimulation may be used to distract one's attention from the core emotional or situational issues which, when contemplated, induce negative mood. This assumes that negative affect is being kept at bay by the distraction. Baumeister and Heatherton[19] described the process as follows, "the source of emotional distress is not present in the immediate situation, but is highly available in memory (eg, immediately after a major rejection or failure experience). Under such circumstances, people seek to distract themselves to prevent thinking about the upsetting event" (p. 5). This pattern seems more relevant to episodic use of sexual behavior, than typical recurring patterns of out-of-control sexuality.
3. The tendency for sexual interest and arousability to be increased in negative mood states characterized by increased arousal (such as anxiety or stress) may result from "excitation transfer".[20] For most individuals, negative affect inhibits sexual responsiveness. But persons prone to out-of-control sexual behavior might not experience this inhibition. Instead excitation may occur and lead to establishment of learned or even conditioned associations between negative mood and sexual arousal. This pattern is most likely to be manifested in solitary

or masturbatory patterns of behavior. Transfer of the anxiety or stress into sexual arousal creates a strong incentive to pursue sexual release through orgasm. The subsequent recognition of this as a recurring and out-of-control pattern induces further negative mood. In some individuals, depression can be associated with anxiety, and the potential for combining patterns 1 and 3.

A key question is why some individuals have the capacity for these atypical and potentially problematic interactions between mood and sexuality and others do not. In our previous studies, we found a negative correlation between MSQ score and age in heterosexual men, which probably means that such paradoxical patterns are more common in younger men and lessen as they get older. When does such an association becomes established? A paradoxical mood/sexuality relationship may develop during childhood or early adolescence as a consequence of early experiences that combine sexual response with negative mood, such as child sexual abuse or induced guilt about masturbation. This possibility would not be difficult to test with retrospective research.

Coleman[21] has postulated that the predisposition to use substances or behaviors to alleviate emotional pain may reflect an "intimacy dysfunction," which could result from child sexual abuse or neglect. An early established pattern of increased sexual arousal and interest in association with negative mood could interfere with normal sexual development, creating a barrier to the incorporation of one's sexuality into close, intimate sexual relationships. In our study of sexual risk taking in heterosexual men,[13] we found that men in exclusive, monogamous relationships had lower MSQ scores and were less likely to report this paradoxical pattern.

IMPAIRED INHIBITION OF SEXUAL AROUSAL

Goodman,[22] in his review of the theoretical basis of sexual addiction, proposed impaired behavioral inhibition as one causal factor. The Kinsey Institute's Dual Control Model postulates that sexual arousal depends on a balance between excitatory and inhibitory systems in the brain, and that individuals vary in their propensity for either sexual excitation or sexual inhibition.[23] Inhibition of sexual response is, according to this perspective, an adaptive mechanism across species. The concept of low propensity for sexual inhibition has already proved useful in explaining some aspects of high-risk sexual behavior.[13,14] In our sex addicts study,[15] we found that sex addicts scored significantly higher on propensity for sexual excitation (SES), but did not differ from controls in two measures of proneness to inhibition (SIS1, inhibition due to the threat of performance failure, and SIS2, inhibition due to the threat of performance consequences).[24] This comparison needs to be replicated in a larger sample before we dismiss this aspect of sexual inhibition as irrelevant to out-of-control sexual behavior, keeping in mind that the questions used to measure SIS1 and SIS2 might not capture the type of inhibition most relevant in this case.

The neurobiology and psychopharmacology of sexual inhibition is complex,[25] but serotonin is clearly involved. Kafka[10] proposed that a dysregulation of central monoamine function is fundamental to out-of-control sexual behavior. Goodman[22] reminded us, however, of the difficulties in localizing complex effects within the central nervous system, or specific to particular neurotransmitters. Thus our use of the Dual Control Model has been based on conceptual systems in the brain, defined in terms of function rather than specific neurotransmitter mediation or anatomic localization.[25] There is, however, a clear need for well-designed, controlled studies of SSRI treatment for men and women with out-of-control sexual behavior, in which groups are carefully selected and matched for indicators of impaired inhibition as well as other behavioral characteristics.

Increased understanding of the genetics of neurotransmitters is creating new possibilities for explaining individual differences. Do those who develop out-of-control patterns of sexual behavior have lower levels of serotonin transporter gene markers?[26] Another new approach to the study of central inhibitory mechanisms is the use of brain imaging (eg, Stoléru and colleagues[27]), which shows that certain areas of the brain are deactivated during response to sexual stimuli. Such deactivation, at least in some areas such as the temporal lobe, may indicate the reduction of inhibitory tone. These techniques are still at an early stage of development, particularly for exploring complex processes such as sexual arousal. But it could be informative to compare the patterns of brain activity in response to sexual stimuli in individuals with 'out of control' sexual behavior and normal controls.

Of possible relevance to neurophysiological inhibition, is the problem of "persistent genital arousal disorder," which has only recently received attention in the literature. It appears to be a uniquely female problem and this in itself requires explanation. One of the two women in our sex addicts study[15] fit this diagnosis, describing herself masturbating as "like a gerbil on a wheel."

Leiblum and colleagues[28,29] identified at least two subtypes of persistent genital arousal, referred to as PGAD and non-PGAD. The PGAD group was more likely to report their genital response and arousal as continuous, overwhelming, and distressing, whereas the non-PGAD group sometimes reported pleasurable feelings associated with their genital response, and felt less distressed by it overall. In a further Web-based survey, 76 women with PGAD were significantly more likely to be depressed, to report panic attacks, and to monitor their physical sensations in an obsessive-compulsive manner than the 48 women in the non-PGAD category. The association between genital response and negative mood is clearly relevant to this phenomenon, but not necessarily different from that experienced by men.

Two gender differences in sexual response may be relevant, however. First, women have much less refractory inhibition after orgasm than men; thus, orgasms are less likely to have a limiting effect. (It would be interesting to study whether the post-ejaculatory refractory period in men with out-of-control sexual behavior differs from healthy controls.) Another uniquely female aspect of genital response is the 'automatic' increase in vaginal blood flow in the presence of any sexually relevant stimulus, whether or not the woman finds the stimulus appealing.[30] This response may initiate a process of monitoring in certain women, leading to the augmentation and persistence of the response because of the impact of negative emotions. As yet, however, we can only speculate about the explanation of PGAD, which could certainly lead to out-of-control sexual behavior, particularly masturbation, in women.

The concept of inhibition, however, presents us with a fundamental challenge. To what extent does it involve relatively automatic neurophysiological processes or alternatively, conscious mechanisms of self-regulation? To what extent is out-of-control or unregulated sexual behavior similar to other out-of-control behaviors like binge eating or overspending? Or is this problem peculiar to control of sexual response? Let us next consider the more cognitive concept of self-regulation.

FAILURES OF SELF-REGULATION

Baumeister and Heatherton[19] provide a useful theoretical approach to failures of self-regulation, which they describe as a multifaceted process that can break down in several different ways. Although their theoretical analysis was not developed to specifically address regulation of sexual behavior, it is relevant in several respects. They describe three components of self-regulation: (1) standards, (2) monitoring, and (3) the operative phase of regulation. Standards are of interest, in particular the dilemmas strict standards can impose, undermining regulation in the process. For five of the male sex addicts in our study,[15] religion was very important. For such individuals, the unquestionable moral unacceptability of most types of sexual behavior conflicts with their sexual impulses, undermining any sensible pattern of regulated sexual behavior. For example, for an individual who believes masturbation to be evil, and who has strong impulses to masturbate on the Internet, a regulated pattern of masturbation is not an acceptable alternative, although for most people this can be a responsible way of dealing with their sexual needs. According to Coleman,[21] highly restrictive sexual attitudes can result in inability to conform, starting off a cycle of guilt, pain, and compulsivity.

Self-monitoring is fundamental to effective self-regulation. Baumeister and Heatherton[19] see relevant effects of alcohol use, as well as fatigue and stress, as impairing normal monitoring. Called "alcohol myopia" by Steele and Josephs[31] and "euphoric recall" by others, it occurs when intoxication causes attention to focus on the positive, sexually arousing, or rewarding aspects of the situation and away from negative consequences and associated inhibition of arousal. We have postulated that sexual arousal per se may also have this effect.[32]

There is another way to conceptualize this aspect of monitoring, which Baumeister and Heatherton[19] described as "transcendence" or focusing one's awareness beyond the immediate situation, so that distal concerns or consequences are kept in mind. In our sex addicts study,[15] we unexpectedly found indications of a dissociative tendency that could contribute to out-of-control behavior by undermining, if not eliminating, this "transcendence." When asked to describe a typical state of mind while acting out, 14 (45%) gave descriptions suggestive of some degree of dissociation. Here are illustrative examples, each from a different subject: "…an overpowering drive…nothing else is under consideration"; "…numb, completely zoning out, not present, not conscious of reality"; "…trancelike state…kills time and pain…numb like a dream"; "when I'm sexually aroused, I click out"; "…feel detached from what is happening"; "…like a drug to numb out." Such explanations may be post hoc justifications, but dissociation has not been explored in the relevant literature and warrants closer study. Do people with out-of-control sexual behavior show more dissociative tendencies in general?

These general aspects of self-regulation, about which there is a substantial literature,[33] are clearly relevant to out-of-control sexual behavior.

OUT-OF-CONTROL SEXUAL BEHAVIOR AS AN ADDICTION

Another explanatory mechanism proposed by Goodman[22] was "aberrant function of the motivational reward system." As yet we can say little about the relevance of reward and incentive mechanisms to out-of-control sexual behavior. But some changes in sensitivity of the incentive reward system may occur as an out-of-control pattern becomes established, similar to changes associated with chronic use of drugs of addiction[34] and possibly with various behavioral addictions.[35] Brain imaging offers possibilities for future research on this issue, as demonstrated in a study of gambling.[36] At this stage of our knowledge, however, the concept of "sexual addiction" is best seen as an analogy, which may be useful at least for some individuals, when used in therapeutic programs.

"OUT-OF-CONTROL" SEXUAL BEHAVIOR AS AN OBSESSIVE-COMPULSIVE DISORDER

The term "compulsive" is often used in this literature without any indication of whether it relates to the compulsivity that is part of obsessive-compulsive disorder. According to the DSM-IV, out-of-control sexual behavior is excluded from the obsessive-compulsive (OCD) category on the grounds that "the person usually derives pleasure from the activity and may wish to resist it only because of its deleterious consequences".[37] Compulsive thoughts of OCD-type often do have sexual content, but are typically accompanied by negative mood and no sexual arousal. We would anticipate that most people with obsessive-compulsive personalities combined with a propensity for mood disorders would experience a decline in sexual arousability during negative mood states, as is the case for most people. But exceptions are likely. Warwick and Salkovskis[38] described two men whose obsessive-compulsive symptoms included intrusive sexual thoughts accompanied by penile erection. The awareness of the erection intensified their anxiety, thus reinforcing the process. This may mean that when some individuals' obsessive-compulsive tendencies are combined with a low propensity for inhibition and/or high propensity for excitation of sexual response, an atypical, sexualized type of compulsive behavioral pattern results. If so, one would expect to find evidence of other obsessive-compulsive phenomena in such individuals. A few studies have looked for evidence of obsessive-compulsive personality among sex addicts, usually finding a small minority in this category (eg, Black and colleagues,[7] 15%; Shapira and colleagues,[39] 15%).

Obsessive-compulsive phenomena, in psychiatric thinking, are characterized by their ego-dystonic nature, usually manifested by some attempt to resist compulsive urges. In our sex addicts study,[15] subjects were asked whether they tried to resist the urge to "act out" or whether at the time it was something they genuinely wanted to do. Eleven men and one woman said that they tried to resist, but most did not give a convincing description of resistance (eg, "I tell myself not to do it, but I do it anyway"). The two most convincing accounts of resistance were from men with obsessive-compulsive personalities. In both cases the sexual acting-out was masturbation. One man had intrusive thoughts about teenage boys, or a compulsion to look at pictures of them. This was associated with considerable guilt and resistance, so he masturbated to achieve a very transient calming effect, followed quickly by renewed guilt and depression. His resistance was to the intrusive thought about boys rather than the masturbation. The other man described ruminative preoccupation with sexual thoughts, which led to masturbation followed by the need to shower because of the "dirtiness" of the act.

Thus, some forms of out-of-control sexual behavior can be appropriately regarded as atypical obsessive-compulsive phenomena, but this clearly applies to a small minority: 7% in our study and approximately 15% in other studies that have assessed it.

SUMMARY

At this stage of our knowledge, it seems reasonable to assume that out-of-control sexual behavior results from a variety of etiological mechanisms associated with different behavioral patterns that share Goodman's[22] two key features of addictive behavior: (1) a recurrent failure to control the sexual behavior; and (2) continuation of the behavior despite harmful consequences. Any overriding definition relevant to clinical management seems premature until we better understand the various patterns and their likely determinants. The concepts of "compulsivity" and "addiction" may have explanatory value in some cases, but are not helpful when used as general terms for this class of behavior problem. Stein and colleagues[11] suggested that, in these circumstances, we use the term "hypersexuality." In my opinion, out-of-control sexual behavior or "impulse control disorders" as proposed by Barth and Kinder[2] are more appropriate nonspecific terms because they focus on the issue of control rather than on high levels of sexuality. A number of clinically relevant and researchable hypotheses need to be addressed in further research, which hopefully will lead to more etiologically or therapeutically relevant subcategories of out-of-control sexual behavior.

REFERENCES

1. Rinehart NJ, McCabe MP. Hypersexuality: psychopathology or normal variant of sexuality? Sexual and Marital Therapy 1997;12(1):45–60.
2. Barth RJ, Kinder BN. The mislabeling of sexual impulsivity. J Sex Marital Ther 1987;13:15–23.
3. Gold SN, Heffner CL. Sexual addiction: many conceptions, minimal data. Clin Psychol Rev 1998;18(8):367–81.
4. Daneback K, Cooper A, Mansson S-A. An Internet study of cybersex participants. Arch Sex Behav 2005;34:321–8.
5. Cooper A, editor. Sex & the Internet: a guidebook for clinicians. New York: Brunner-Routledge; 2002.
6. Raviv M. Personality characteristics of sexual addicts and pathological gamblers. J Gambl Stud 1993;9:17–30.
7. Black DW, Kehrberg LLD, Flumerfelt DL, et al. Characteristics of 36 subjects reporting compulsive sexual behavior. Am J Psychiatry 1997;154(2):243–9.
8. Quadland MC. Compulsive sexual behavior: definition of a problem and an approach to treatment. J Sex Marital Ther 1985;11:121–32.
9. Fedoroff JP. Serotonergic drug treatment of deviant sexual interests. Annals of Sex Research 1993;6:105–21.
10. Kafka MP. A monoamine hypothesis for the patho-physiology of paraphilic disorders. Arch Sex Behav 1997;26(4):343–57.
11. Stein DJ, Hollander E, Anthony DT, et al. Serotonergic medications for sexual obsessions, sexual addictions, and paraphilias. J Clin Psychiatry 1992;53(8):267–71.
12. Mustanski B, Bancroft J. Sexual dysfunction. In: Gorwood P, Hamon M, editors. Psychopharmacogenetics. New York: Springer; 2006. p. 479–94.
13. Bancroft J, Janssen E, Carnes L, et al. Sexual activity and risk-taking in young heterosexual men: the relevance of sexual arousability, mood and sensation seeking. J Sex Res 2004;41:181–92.
14. Bancroft J, Janssen E, Strong D, et al. Sexual risk taking in gay men: the relevance of sexual arousability, mood and sensation seeking. Arch Sex Behav 2003;32:555–72.
15. Bancroft J, Vukadinovic Z. Sexual addiction, sexual compulsivity, sexual impulsivity or what? Towards a theoretical model. J Sex Res 2004;41:225–34.
16. Bancroft J, Janssen E, Strong D, et al. The relation between mood and sexuality in heterosexual men. Arch Sex Behav 2003;32:217–30.
17. Bancroft J, Janssen E, Strong D, et al. The relation between mood and sexuality in gay men. Arch Sex Behav 2003;32:231–42.
18. Lykins AD, Janssen E, Graham CA. The relationship between negative mood and sexuality in heterosexual college women and men. J Sex Res 2006;43:136–43.
19. Baumeister RF, Heatherton TF. Self-regulation failure: an overview. Psychological Inquiry 1996;7(1):1–15.

20. Zillman D. Transfer of excitation in emotional behavior. In: Cacioppo JT, Petty RE, editors. Social psychophysiology: a sourcebook. New York: Guilford Press; 1983. p. 215–40.
21. Coleman E. Sexual compulsion vs. sexual addiction: the debate continues. SIECUS Rep 1986 July;7–11.
22. Goodman A, et al. Sexual addiction. In: Lowinson JH, Ruiz P, Millman RB, editors. Substance abuse: a comprehensive textbook. Philadelphia: Williams & Wilkins; 1997. p. 340–54.
23. Bancroft J, Janssen E. The dual control model of male sexual response: a theoretical approach to centrally mediated erectile dysfunction. Neurosci Biobehav Rev 2000;24:571–9.
24. Janssen E, Vorst H, Finn P, et al. The sexual inhibition (SIS) and sexual excitation (SES) scales: I. Measuring sexual inhibition and excitation proneness in men. J Sex Res 2002;39:114–26.
25. Bancroft J. Central inhibition of sexual response in the male: a theoretical perspective. Neurosci Biobehav Rev 1999;23:763–84.
26. Lesch KP, Bengel D, Heils A, et al. Association of anxiety-related traits with a polymorphism in the serotonin transporter gene regulatory region. Science 1996;274: 1527–31.
27. Stoléru S, Grégoire MC, Gérard D, et al. Neuroanatomical correlates of visually evoked sexual arousal in human males. Arch Sex Behav 1999;28:1–21.
28. Leiblum S, Seehuus M, Brown C. Persistent genital arousal: disordered or normative aspect of female sexual response. J Sex Med 2007;4:680–9.
29. Leiblum S, Seehuus M, Goldmeier D, et al. Psychological, medical and pharmacological correlates or persistent genital arousal disorder. J Sex Med 2007;4:1358–66.
30. Laan E, Everaerd W. Determinants of sexual arousal: psychophysiological theory and data. Annual Review of Sex Research 1995;6:32–76.
31. Steele CM, Josephs RA. Alcohol myopia: its prized and dangerous effects. Am Psychol 1990;45:921–33.
32. Strong DA, Bancroft J, Carnes LA, et al. The impact of sexual arousal on sexual risk taking: a qualitative study. J Sex Res 2005;42:185–91.
33. Baumeister RF, Heatherton TF, Tice DM. Losing control: how and why people fail at self-regulation. San Diego (CA): Academic Press; 1994.
34. Robinson TE, Berridge KC. The neural basis of drug craving: an incentive sensitization theory of addiction. Brain Res Brain Res Rev 1993;18:247–91.
35. Holden C. "Behavioral addictions": do they exist? Science 2001;294:980–2.
36. Breiter HC, Aharon I, Kahneman D, et al. Functional imaging of neural responses to expectancy and experience of monetary gains and losses. Neuron 2001;20: 619–39.
37. American Psychiatric Association. Diagnostic and statistical manual of mental disorders. (text rev). 4th edition. Washington, DC: American Psychiatric Association; 2000. p. 422.
38. Warwick HMC, Salkovskis PM. Unwanted erections in obsessive-compulsive disorder. Br J Psychiatry 1990;157:919–21.
39. Shapira NA, Goldsmith TD, Keck PE, et al. Psychiatric features of individuals with problematic Internet use. J Affect Disord 2000;57:267–72.

Epidemiology, Prevalence, and Natural History of Compulsive Sexual Behavior

John M. Kuzma, MD[a], Donald W. Black, MD[b],*

KEYWORDS

- Impulse control disorders • Compulsive sexual behavior
- Sexual disorders

Charles, a 37-year-old married man, sought psychiatric evaluation after being suspended from work for viewing Internet pornography. Remote monitoring of his Internet use showed that he spent as many as 6 hours each day viewing pornographic Web sites. He masturbated up to 6 times daily while at work. This behavior led to poor work productivity, which prompted increased scrutiny from supervisors, and his eventual suspension.

Charles had a long history of compulsive masturbation, which he claimed was a way to comfort himself during periods of depression and anxiety. He preferred fetish Web sites, which led him to masturbate. Viewing the Web site was closely linked to his sexual arousal, and he reported that he did not obtain sexual release from masturbation alone. He claimed to view pornography at work because his wife had demanded he remove computers from their home due to his uncontrolled sexual behavior. He even left his home at night to access the Internet at work and masturbate.

He reported having a troubled childhood with emotionally distant and verbally abusive parents, but there was no history of physical or sexual abuse. He began to masturbate when he entered puberty at age 12, and by age 14 was masturbating several times daily. At school, as at work later in life, he would masturbate in the restroom. After graduating from high school he briefly attended college before dropping out because of poor academic performance.

Poor productivity and frequent absenteeism characterized Charles' work performance. He had never held a job for more than 2 years. He had been married twice and had three children. His first wife sought a divorce because she could not tolerate his sexually compulsive behavior, and his second wife had recently left for the same

[a] HealthPartners Regions Behavioral Health, 640 Jackson Street, St. Paul, MN 55110, USA
[b] Department of Psychiatry, Psychiatry Research/2-126b MEB, University of Iowa Roy J. and Lucille A. Carver College of Medicine, Iowa City, IA 52242, USA
* Corresponding author.
E-mail address: donald-black@uiowa.edu (D. Black).

Psychiatr Clin N Am 31 (2008) 603–611
doi:10.1016/j.psc.2008.06.005
0193-953X/08/$ – see front matter © 2008 Elsevier Inc. All rights reserved.

reason. He denied engaging in sexual relations with persons other than his wives; never had a homosexual experience; and denied exhibitionism, voyeurism, or other paraphilic behaviors. He had seen several therapists over the years, usually in the context of marital discord, and had sought psychiatric treatment for depression and anxiety. A psychiatrist once prescribed fluoxetine for depression, but Charles discontinued the drug after taking it less than a week, and dropped out of therapy after two sessions. He never disclosed his sexual compulsion to any clinician.

INTRODUCTION

Compulsive sexual behavior (CSB) has been a subject of interest in both the scientific and general literature.[1] Despite this high level of interest, there is ongoing debate about its core features and its relationship to other psychiatric disorders.[2] The general consensus is that CSB is characterized by inappropriate or excessive sexual cognitions or behaviors that lead to subjective distress or impaired functioning in one or more important life domains.[3]

CSB can be divided into paraphilic and nonparaphilic subtypes.[4] The former involves pathological sexual behaviors, while the later involves conventional sexual behaviors taken to extremes.[4] In DSM-IV-TR, eight specific paraphilias (**Table 1**) are enumerated.[5] Other forms of paraphilia are best diagnosed as "paraphilic disorder not otherwise specified." There is no DSM-IV-TR category that corresponds to the nonparaphilic forms of CSB, although the category "sexual disorder not otherwise specified" can be used.[5]

Research into CSB has been hampered by inadequate sampling methods and the lack of reliable diagnostic criteria. Operational criteria, such as those proposed by Goodman,[6] Black,[1] and Stein and colleagues[7] may help investigators by providing

Table 1		
DSM-IV-TR nomenclature for CSB-related disorders		
I. Paraphilic		
Name	Urges/Behavior	ICD-9 Code
Exhibitionism	Exposing one's genitals to strangers	302.4
Fetishism	Use of nonliving objects	302.81
Frotteurism	Rubbing against a nonconsenting person	302.89
Pedophilia	Sexual acts with a prepubescent child	302.2
Masochism	Experiencing pain and suffering	302.83
Sadism	Inflicting pain and suffering	302.84
Transvestic	Fetishism cross-dressing	302.3
Voyeurism	Observing sexual activity of strangers	302.82
Paraphilia, NOS	Other abnormal sexual urges or behaviors	302.9
II. Nonparaphilic		
Sexual Disorder, NOS	Culturally acceptable sexual urges and behavior to excess.	302.9

Abbreviations: CSB, compulsive sexual behavior; DSM, Diagnostic and Statistical Manual; NOS, not otherwise specified.

Data from American Psychiatric Association. Task Force on DSM-IV. Diagnostic and statistical manual of mental disorders: DSM-IV-TR. 4th edition. Washington, DC: American Psychiatric Association; 2000.

greater specificity for the diagnosis. Research is also limited in part by the sensitive nature of sex, as well as ongoing debate about the theoretical underpinnings of the disorder.[8] Some investigators have observed that the complex role of sex in our culture makes it difficult to consider CSB as a discrete psychiatric disorder rather than a deviation from cultural norms.[8] Others, while acknowledging the complicated nature of sex, have focused on the adverse consequences of CSB and considered impairment a key element of the disorder.[1]

PREVALENCE

The estimated prevalence of CSB ranges from 3% to 6% in the general adult population of the United States.[9,10] These are rough estimates because the private nature of sex and the continuing stigma involved with these behaviors likely leads to underreporting due to embarrassment or shame.[3] This may skew the clinical picture of CSB because perhaps only the most severe cases are seen.

Data on the frequency of orgasm may correlate with CSB prevalence and serve as an indicator of prevalence. Kinsey and colleagues[11] developed the concept of the total sexual outlet (TSO), defined as a number of orgasms achieved through any means during a designate week. They found that 7.6% of men up to age 30 had an average TSO of ≥ 7 for at least 5 years, primarily through masturbation. The median TSO was 2.14 for that age group, and 1.99 for all men.[11] Atwood and Gagnon[12] reported that 5% of high school–age boys and 3% of college-age white males masturbated at least once daily. Lauman[13] reported that 34% of men between 18 and 25 years old masturbated once per week, 15% two to six times weekly, 2% daily, and 1% more than once daily in the past year.

Examining these and other data, Kafka[14] suggested that ≥ 7 weekly orgasms over six consecutive months could be used to define hypersexual behavior, a concept that corresponds to CSB. Kinsey and colleagues[11] criticized the notion of high-frequency sexual behavior as being inherently pathologic. Others have agreed, and have focused on the subjective distress and psychosocial dysfunction, not frequency of orgasm.[1] A study from Sweden suggested that simple frequency of sexual activity is an insufficient metric for CSB.[15] Ironically, they noted that high-frequency sexual behavior *with a stable partner* is associated with better psychological functioning, while frequent solitary or impersonal sexual behavior correlated with comorbid psychiatric disorder and psychosocial dysfunction. Thus, a high frequency of orgasms is not by itself pathological.

A study of 204 consecutively admitted psychiatric inpatients found a 4.4% current prevalence and 4.9% lifetime prevalence of CSB.[16] The authors noted that the lack of notable difference between current and lifetime prevalence suggests this disorder may be chronic when untreated.

GENDER DISTRIBUTION

While no community studies address this issue, nearly all pertinent clinical reports show a male preponderance (**Table 2**).[8,17] For example, in a study of 36 persons with self-identified CSB, only 22% were women.[18] Other studies of CSB have examined only men, representing a clear selection bias.[1] Reports from centers that treat "sexual addictions" also found a male preponderance. Along these lines, Carnes and Delmonico[19] reported that 80% of 290 persons surveyed were male. Similarly, 84% of 76 married persons attending a 12-step program for sex addicts were male.[20] When CSB is examined dimensionally, men have more symptoms as well. Dodge and

Table 2
Demographic features and lifetime psychiatric comorbidity in persons with CSB

Subjects	Black et al[18] (n = 36)	Kafka and Rentky[25] (n = 26)	Raymond et al[17] (n = 25)
Source	Advertisement	Outpatient clinic	Advertisement
Female	22%	0%	8%
Age, mean, y	27	34	38
Age at onset, mean, y	18	—	—
Diagnostic assessment used	DIS/PDQ-R/SIDP-R	"Intake questionnaire"	SCID/SCID-II
Mood disorders	39%	81%	71%
Anxiety disorders	50%	46%	96%
Eating disorders	11%	0%	8%
Substance use disorders	64%	46%	71%
Impulse control disorders	—	—	—
Pathological gambling	11%	0%	4%
Kleptomania	14%	4%	13%
Trichotillomania	3%	0%	—
IED	3%	4%	13%
Pyromania	8%	0%	—
Compulsive buying	14%	—	—
Any ICD	—	—	38%
Paraphilia	—	—	8%
Sexual dysfunction	—	—	46%
Any Axis II disorder	44%	—	46%

Abbreviations: CSB, compulsive sexual behavior; DIS, Diagnostic Interview Schedule; ICD, impulse control disorder; IED, intermittent explosive disorder; PDQ-R, Personality Diagnostic Questionnaire-Revised; SCID, Structured Interview for DSM-IV Axis I Disorders; SCID-II, Structured Interview for DSM-IV Axis II Disorders; SIDP-R, Structured Interview for DSM-III-R Personality Disorders.

colleagues[21] reported a statistically significant difference in mean Sexual Compulsivity Scale (SCS) scores for men (1.64) and women (1.33). The SCS is a reliable and valid scale used to study populations at risk for dangerous sexual behaviors[22] and has more recently been used in examining sexual behaviors in college students.[21]

There may be differences in the way CSB presents in men and women.[4] Evidence suggests that men are more likely to have compulsive masturbation, engage in paraphilias, pay for sex, or engage in anonymous sex.[8] Women are more likely to engage in fantasy sex (eg, seductive behavior leading to multiple affairs/relationships) or sado-masochism, or to use sex as a business. Women with CSB are more likely to experience emotional attachments, for example presenting as a series of multiple failed or dangerous relationships,[3] and may refer to themselves as "love addicts." The study of Black and colleagues[18] found that men with CSB had a mean of 59 sexual partners in the previous 5 years compared with 8 for women; this, too, suggests that women are less focused on physical aspects of sex than are men.[18]

CSB may be more common in gay and bisexual men.[23] A recent study examining psychiatric comorbidity in pathological gamblers is relevant; Grant and Potenza[24] found that 59% of gay or bisexual subjects had a lifetime prevalence of CSB as compared with 14.5% of heterosexual males.

NATURAL HISTORY

There are few data regarding the natural history of CSB. Nonetheless, evidence suggests that CSB has an onset in adolescence, with paraphilic behaviors frequently occurring earlier than nonparaphilic behaviors,[18,25] and that for most the disorder is chronic or episodic. However, these same studies also show a long delay before their subjects sought treatment, perhaps because of the stigma that persons with CSB experience.

CSB has been characterized as a progressive, multiphase illness that grows more intense the longer it is untreated.[26,27] In the first phase, *preoccupation*, a person develops sexual thoughts and urges. The next phase, *ritualization*, involves the development of an idiosyncratic routine that prompts the sexual behavior. The third phase, *gratification*, involves the sexual behavior itself. The fourth phase, *despair*, is characterized by feelings of guilt, powerlessness, and isolation, all of which fuel the tension underlying CSB and prompt the person to repeat the cycle. Bergner[27] also noted that CSB patients follow a recurrent pattern in their behavior and argued that fantasy scenarios are derived from early experiences of degradation. He suggests that CSB represents an internalized attempt to recover from the trauma of that degradation.

CLINICAL DESCRIPTION

In their sample of 36 persons with CSB, Black and colleagues[18] reported that 92% were obsessed with sexual urges and fantasies, or that they were overly sexually active. Fifteen subjects (42%) admitted that their repetitive fantasies were out of control or caused subjective distress. Of these individuals, most reported that they had made unsuccessful attempts to resist acting on their fantasies (eg, making pacts or New Year's resolutions), and felt ashamed after having a fantasy. These investigators also found that three quarters of the subjects abused drugs or alcohol while engaging in their compulsive behaviors, perhaps disinhibiting them sufficiently to promote the activity, to enhance their pleasure, or to numb their sense of shame. When asked what they disliked about the CSB, they reported the lack of control and its time-consuming nature. Other concerns involved its cost (eg, prostitutes, pornography), the fact that significant others had been betrayed, losing friends, or experiencing shame. One respondent said the CSB made her "feel like a whore." Nearly two thirds were subjectively distressed by their sexual thoughts or behaviors, and nearly half felt that it caused impairment in important life domains, such as their marriage or important relationships, or that it had affected their work (eg, through intrusive thoughts or from frequent lateness).

In the study of Raymond and colleagues,[17] nearly half the sample reported thoughts of CSB on a daily basis, but most reported spending less than 60 minutes daily experiencing sexual urges. About one third described their sexual thoughts as intrusive, and over two thirds had attempted to resist thoughts and 87% to resist urges. Most indicated that they disliked their compulsive thoughts and behaviors, although for most the behavior led to tension relief and a sense of gratification.

PSYCHIATRIC COMORBIDITY

Psychiatric comorbidity is the rule and not the exception for persons with CSB.[4] Black and colleagues,[18] Kafka and Prentky,[25] and Raymond and colleagues[17] have reported that persons with CSB frequently meet criteria for other psychiatric disorders, especially mood, anxiety, substance use, and personality disorders (see **Table 2**). In these studies, persons with CSB were frequently found to meet criteria for Axis I disorders, and while none used a control group, the figures for Axis I disorders are greater than those from epidemiologic samples. Disorders of impulse control were relatively common in the studies of Black and colleagues[18] and Raymond and colleagues.[17] Grant and Kim[28] reported that pathological gambling may have a special relationship with CSB; of 96 pathological gamblers, 9.4% reported a lifetime history of the disorder. Kafka[29] has also reported an increased prevalence of attention deficit disorder in persons with CSB.

Persons who view CSB as an addiction see it as one of many that a patient might suffer. In a survey of nearly 1000 persons admitted for residential treatment of CSB, Carnes[9] found that 42% reported a history of substance dependence, and 38% stated they had an eating disorder. Carnes and Delmonico[19] reported similar figures in a survey of 290 "recovering sex addicts." In this study, 39% reported an alcohol or drug dependency, 57% "codependency," 36% an eating disorder, 26% tobacco addiction, 21% caffeine addiction, 28% compulsive working, 23% compulsive spending, 4% compulsive gambling, and 12% other forms of compulsive behavior.

Kafka and Prentky[25] observed that many persons with CSB manifest multiple paraphilias or nonparaphilic forms of CSB. For example, a man who is heterosexually promiscuous might also use pornography and compulsively masturbate. In the study of Black and colleagues,[18] overlap was seen among the nonparaphilic forms of CSB, although this was not seen with the paraphilia, perhaps because of the reluctance of subjects to disclose potentially illegal behaviors. While Raymond and colleagues[17] reported that nearly half of their subjects had sexual dysfunction (mainly male erectile disorder or inhibited female orgasm), there were few additional paraphilias. On the other hand, Grant[30] found that among 25 men with exhibitionism, 28% met general criteria for CSB, suggesting great overlap of these conditions.

Axis II disorders are also common in persons with CSB, although there is no evidence for a "CSB personality." Black and colleagues[18] reported that 44% of their sample met criteria for a personality disorder based on a consensus of two instruments, most commonly the histrionic, paranoid, and obsessive-compulsive types. In this study, cluster A disorders were found in 15%, cluster B disorders in 29%, and cluster C disorders in 24%. More recently, Raymond and colleagues[17] reported that 46% of 25 persons with CSB had a personality disorder. Like Black and colleagues, they did not find evidence of a relationship to any particular personality disorder. Cluster A disorders were found in 20%, cluster B disorders 20%, and cluster C disorders 39%. Raymond and colleagues[17] make the point that in these samples, cluster B and C disorders have nearly the same frequency, which may be counterintuitive because one might expect that persons with CSB would tend to "act out," suggesting the presence of an antisocial, borderline, or histrionic personality disorder. Yet, these investigators suggest that many individuals with CSB are anxious persons who likely have trouble establishing intimacy. Drawing on his clinical experience, Carnes[9] reported that the cluster B personality traits were common in persons with CSB, with men frequently displaying antisocial traits, and women more commonly displaying dependent, borderline, and hysterical personality traits.

MEDICAL COMORBIDITY

CSB patients frequently engage in high-risk sexual behavior that places them at risk for sexually transmitted diseases (STDs) or physical trauma such as bruising.[31] Physical injuries can result from high-risk sexual behaviors or sadomasochistic activity.

In women, unwanted pregnancies can occur, as can complications from an abortion. A study of a predominately African American population at an urban clinic for sexually transmitted disease found that patients with an SCS score more than 80% above the mean were four times as likely to have been diagnosed with multiple STDs than those scoring 80% below the mean.[31] A similar association between CSB and unsafe sexual practices was observed in a population of college students.[21] A study of 294 HIV-positive men and women found that those with CSB reported more acts of unprotected vaginal and anal intercourse with HIV-negative partners than those who did not.[32]

FAMILY HISTORY AND RISK FACTORS

There are no family studies of CSB. Nonetheless, uncontrolled data suggest that substance misuse and mental illness are common in relatives. Schneider and Schneider[20] reported that in a survey of 75 recovering sex addicts, 40% reported at least one parent as chemically dependent; 36% reported that one or both parents were sex addicts; 33% reported that one or both parents had an eating disorder; and 7% reported that one parent was a compulsive gambler. A small family history study that may be relevant to CSB found an increased rate of pedophilia among relatives of patients with pedophilia (19%) versus relatives of healthy controls (3%).[33] This has led some to suggest that CSB and other paraphilias may have a genetic diathesis.[3]

A history of childhood sexual abuse (CSA) is thought by some to be a risk factor for CSB. In a survey of self-identified persons with CSB nearly 80% also endorsed CSA.[19] Other researchers have reported much lower rates; for example Black and colleagues[18] who reported a rate of 31%, and Kafka and Prentky[25] a rate of 28%.

SUMMARY

Research into CSB is hindered by the lack of a generally accepted definition and reliable and valid assessment tools. Despite these limitations, evidence indicates that CSB is relatively common in the general adult population, causes substantial personal distress, and is a source of significant psychosocial disability. CSB appears to begin early in life, to have a male preponderance, and to run a chronic or episodic course. It is also commonly associated with psychiatric comorbidity, typically mood, anxiety, substance use, and personality disorders. Further research is needed to better our understanding of the disorder and improve our ability to develop specific interventions.

REFERENCES

1. Black DW. Compulsive sexual behavior: a review. Journal of Practical Psychiatry and Behavioral Health 1998;4(7):219–29.
2. Mick TM, Hollander E. Impulsive-compulsive sexual behavior. CNS Spectr 2006; 11(12):944–55.
3. Black DW. The epidemiology and phenomenology of compulsive sexual behavior. CNS Spectr 2000;5(1):26–35.
4. Coleman E, Raymond N, McBean A. Assessment and treatment of compulsive sexual behavior. Minn Med 2003;86(7):42–7.
5. American Psychiatric Association. American Psychiatric Association. Task Force on DSM-IV. Diagnostic and statistical manual of mental disorders: DSM-IV-TR. 4th edition. Washington, DC: American Psychiatric Association; 2000.

6. Goodman A. Diagnosis and treatment of sexual addiction. J Sex Marital Ther 1993;19(3):225–51.

7. Stein DJ, Black DW, Pienaar W. Sexual disorders not otherwise specified: compulsive, addictive, or impulsive? CNS Spectr 2000;5(1):60–4.

8. Bancroft J, Vukadinovic Z. Sexual addiction, sexual compulsivity, sexual impulsivity, or what? Toward a theoretical model. J Sex Res 2004;41(3):225–34.

9. Carnes P. Don't call it love: recovery from sexual addiction. New York: Bantam Publishing; 1991.

10. Coleman E. Is your patient suffering from compulsive sexual behavior? Psychiatr Ann 1992;22:320–5.

11. Kinsey AC, Pomeroy WB, Martin CE. Sexual behavior in the human male. Philadelphia: W.B. Saunders Co.; 1948.

12. Atwood J, Gagnon J. Masturbatory behavior in college youth. J Sex Educ Ther 1987;13:35–42.

13. Laumann EO. The social organization of sexuality: sexual practices in the United States. Chicago: University of Chicago Press; 1994.

14. Kafka MP. Hypersexual desire in males: an operational definition and clinical implications for males with paraphilias and paraphilia-related disorders. Arch Sex Behav 1997;26(5):505–26.

15. Langstrom N, Hanson RK. High rates of sexual behavior in the general population: correlates and predictors. Arch Sex Behav 2006;35(1):37–52.

16. Grant JE, Levine L, Kim D, et al. Impulse control disorders in adult psychiatric inpatients. Am J Psychiatry 2005;162(11):2184–8.

17. Raymond NC, Coleman E, Miner MH. Psychiatric comorbidity and compulsive/impulsive traits in compulsive sexual behavior. Compr Psychiatry 2003;44(5): 370–80.

18. Black DW, Kehrberg LL, Flumerfelt DL, et al. Characteristics of 36 subjects reporting compulsive sexual behavior. Am J Psychiatry 1997;154(2):243–9.

19. Carnes PJ, Delmonico DL. Childhood abuse and multiple addictions: research findings in a sample of self-identified sexual addicts. Sexual Addiction and Compulsivity 1996;3:11.

20. Schneider JP, Schneider BH. Couple recovery from sexual addiction: research findings of a survey of 88 marriages. Sexual Addiction and Compulsivity 1996; 3:111–26.

21. Dodge B, Reece M, Cole SL, et al. Sexual compulsivity among heterosexual college students. J Sex Res 2004;41(4):343–50.

22. Kalichman SC, Rompa D. Sexual sensation seeking and sexual compulsivity scales: reliability, validity, and predicting HIV risk behavior. J Pers Assess 1995;65(3):586–601.

23. Warner J, McKeown F, Griffin M, et al. Rates and predictors of mental illness in gay men, lesbians and bisexual men and women: results from a survey based in England and Wales. Br J Psychiatry 2004;185:479–85.

24. Grant JE, Potenza MN. Sexual orientation of men with pathological gambling: prevalence and psychiatric comorbidity in a treatment-seeking sample. Compr Psychiatry 2006;47(7):515–8.

25. Kafka MP, Prentky R. A comparative study of nonparaphilic sexual addictions and paraphilias in men. J Clin Psychiatry 1992;53(10):345–50.

26. Carnes P. Addiction or compulsion: politics or illness? Sexual addiction and Compulsivity 1996;3:22.

27. Bergner RM. Sexual compulsion as attempted recovery from degradation: theory and therapy. J Sex Marital Ther 2002;28(5):373–87.

28. Grant JE, Kim SW. Comorbidity of impulse control disorders in pathological gamblers. Acta Psychiatr Scand 2003;108(3):203–7.
29. Kafka MP. Paraphilia-related disorders–common, neglected, and misunderstood. Harv Rev Psychiatry 1994;2(1):39–40.
30. Grant JE. Clinical characteristics and psychiatric comorbidity in males with exhibitionism. J Clin Psychiatry 2005;66(11):1367–71.
31. Kalichman SC, Cain D. The relationship between indicators of sexual compulsivity and high risk sexual practices among men and women receiving services from a sexually transmitted infection clinic. J Sex Res 2004;41(3):235–41.
32. Benotsch E, Kalichman SC, Pinkerton SD. Sexual-compulsivity in HIV-positive men and women: prevalence, predictors, and consequences of high risk behaviors. Sexual Addiction and Compulsivity 2001;9(4):9.
33. Gaffney GR, Lurie SF, Berlin FS. Is there familial transmission of pedophilia? J Nerv Ment Dis 1984;172(9):546–8.

Paraphilia from a Dissociative Perspective

Colin A. Ross, MD

KEYWORDS

• Dissociative disorders • Paraphilia • Sexual abuse

Only one study[1] has examined the rates of childhood trauma and dissociative disorders among male sex offenders. There have been no studies in women. The one published study involved only 13 participants who received a structured interview for dissociative disorders, the Dissociative Disorders Interview Schedule.[2] Of the 13 offenders, all interviewed at an inpatient treatment center, 10 (76.9%) had a dissociative disorder of some kind, including 5 (38.5%) with dissociative identity disorder. More studies with larger samples taken from a variety of settings are required before any conclusions can be reached about the prevalence of dissociative disorders among sex offenders, or among individuals with noncriminal paraphilias.

The purpose of this article is to present a clinical model and understanding of paraphilia from a dissociative perspective. Numerous other perspectives are also required to understand the paraphilias.

THE DEFINITION OF DISSOCIATION

Confusion about dissociation can arise because the word has four different meanings.[3] The first meaning of dissociation is a general systems meaning: dissociation is the opposite of association. When two things are associated, they are connected, interacting, and in some sort of relationship with each other. When two things are dissociated, they are disconnected from each other, and not interacting with each other. Dissociations between variables can be partial or complete. Dissociation in this sense is a general phenomenon and occurs in physical chemistry, for instance.

Second, dissociation is a phenomenological term within psychology and psychiatry. Dissociation is measured in scales and structured interviews, such as the Dissociative Experiences Scale (DES),[4] Dissociative Disorders Interview Schedule (DDIS),[2] Structured Clinical Interview for DSM-IV Dissociative Disorders (SCID-D),[5] and Multidimensional Inventory of Dissociation (MID).[6] The reliability and validity of dissociation, and of the dissociative disorders, have been established by a substantial research

The Colin A. Ross Institute for Psychological Trauma, 1701 Gateway, 349, Richardson, TX 75080, USA
E-mail address: rossinst@rossinst.com

Psychiatr Clin N Am 31 (2008) 613–622
doi:10.1016/j.psc.2008.06.008
0193-953X/08/$ – see front matter © 2008 Elsevier Inc. All rights reserved.

literature. The rules for establishing the reliability and validity of dissociation are the same as those for anxiety, depression, and psychosis.

In one study,[7] for example, the DES, DDIS, and SCID-D were administered to 110 general adult psychiatric inpatients. Interviewers administering the two structured interviews, the DDIS and SCID-D, were blind to results of the other interviews. The DES is a 28-item self-report measure that contains an eight-item subscale called the DES-taxon, or DES-T. Taxometric analysis of the scores for the eight DES-T items results in the participant being assigned to one of two dichotomous categories: in the taxon or out of the taxon. Individuals who are in the taxon have chronic, complex dissociative disorders according to the DES-T.

Clinical interviews were conducted on 50 of the participants by a clinician blind to the results of the DES, DDIS, and SCID-D. Each diagnostic method assigned the participant to one of two categories: dissociative identity disorder (DID) or dissociative disorder not otherwise specified (DDNOS), versus no dissociative disorder.

The rates of agreement between the different diagnostic methods using Cohen's kappa were as follows: DDIS-SCID-D 0.74, DDIS-Clinician 0.71, SCID-D-Clinician 0.56, DDIS-DES-T 0.81, SCID-D-DES-T 0.76, and DES-T-Clinician 0.74. The results indicate that individuals can be assigned to the dissociative taxon (having either DID or DDNOS) with reliability and concurrent validity between measures that meets the usual standards for Axis I disorders.[8]

This same report[8] also included a table summarizing 11 studies in seven different countries in which general adult psychiatric inpatients were screened with the DES, then interviewed with either the DDIS or the SCID-D. In all these studies, individuals with prior dissociative disorder diagnoses were excluded. Pooling the studies, the total number of participants was 1644; of these, 15.3% had a dissociative disorder of some kind, including 3.7% with dissociative identity disorder (DID).

The existing research indicates that dissociative disorders are not rare in clinical settings, and can be detected with good reliability and concurrent validity. The second meaning of dissociation is thus supported by a substantial research literature.

The third meaning of dissociation is its use as a technical term in cognitive psychology.[9] For instance, a dissociation between procedural and declarative memory has been demonstrated in numerous experiments involving a wide range of tasks, sensory modalities, and cognitive skills. A typical example is an experiment involving homophonic word pairs, such as *read-reed* and *bare-bear*. These are words that sound the same but have different spellings and meanings.

Participants in an experiment are presented with a list of homophonic word pairs, which they memorize. At a later time they are asked to list as many of the word pairs as they can from memory. The free recall task demonstrates that a number of subjects cannot recall having been exposed to the *read-reed* word pair—in clinical language, they have amnesia for a past experience.

Participants are then asked to write down the name of a tall, tubular plant that grows in marshes. Participants who had *read-reed* on their list of word pairs misspell reed as read more often than participants who did not have *read-reed* in their word lists.

These results demonstrate that prior exposure to the *read-reed* word pair is stored in procedural memory and is affecting behavior, in the absence of declarative memory for the experience. For decades, this effect has been called a dissociation between procedural and declarative memory. Dissociation between procedural and declarative memory is a robustly demonstrated property of normal psychology.

Dissociation in this sense is also an everyday human experience. For instance, one cannot recall the name of an actor—it is "on the tip of my tongue." With repeated recall effort and using associations with other actors and movies, the name is transferred accurately into declarative memory. This is dissociation in the third meaning of the term.

The fourth meaning of dissocation is an intrapsychic defense mechanism. It is important to be clear about which meaning of the word dissociation is intended, otherwise scholars can speak at cross-purposes. For instance, it is true that the intrapsychic defense mechanism of dissociation has not been demonstrated scientifically. The same is true for projection, condensation, and the other classical defense mechanisms. However, the intrapsychic defense mechanism of dissociation is but one possible cause of the phenomenon of dissociation, as measured by the DES, DDIS, SCID-D, and MID.

Dissociation can be valid and reliable at the phenomenological level without the intrapsychic defense mechanism of dissociation being proven or accepted. This is true for all disorders in DSM-IV. There are intrapsychic defense models of schizophrenia, depression, panic disorder, and bulimia, for instance, but the diagnostic reliability and validity of these DSM-IV categories do not depend on the validity of psychoanalytical theory. The reliability and validity of the DSM-IV dissociative disorders, one might say, can be dissociated from the validity of the intrapsychic defense mechanism of dissociation. DSM-IV dissociative disorders are no more dependent on unproven psychoanalytic theories than any other category in the manual.

WHAT DISSOCIATION IS NOT

Dissociation is not a synonym for *repression*. In *Studies on Hysteria*, published in 1895, Breuer and Freud[10] presented a trauma-dissociation model of psychopathology. They described cases of DID and DDNOS with extensive comorbidity and considered the presenting symptoms in adulthood to be causally related to childhood sexual abuse that actually took place. In his 1897 letter to Fleiss, however, Freud[11] repudiated the seduction theory and decided that the incest had never taken place. The memories, he decided, were false memories.

To explain why his women patients were presenting with hysteria and false memories of childhood sexual abuse, Freud developed repression theory. Trauma-dissociation theory assumes, generally and broadly, that the trauma really did take place, although memory is prone to a variety of sources of error. Repression theory assumes that the trauma never happened.

Freud[12] went on to describe two subtypes of repression: *primal repression* and *repression proper*. Primal repression occurs when id impulses and drives that are unacceptable to the ego threaten to emerge into consciousness. They are held down by primal repression. Repression proper occurs when experiences and perceptions of the outside world create conflict in the ego: these are then pushed down into the id for storage. Primal repression has nothing to do with outside events or defenses against them. Only repression proper could potentially be a synonym for the fourth meaning of dissociation.

Even at the level of defense theory, however, repression and dissociation are not the same thing. Freud repudiated dissociation theory; there are no "repression disorders" in DSM-IV; psychoanalysts rarely diagnose dissociative disorders; and repression theory applies when the memories are assumed to be false (to be Oedipal fantasies).

The core difference between the fourth meaning of dissociation and repression is explained best by Hilgard.[13] In his neodissociation theory, he distinguishes between *horizontal splitting* and *vertical splitting*. In horizontal splitting there is a defensive barrier between the id and the ego and the repressed material is held in the id, where it is subject to distortion by primary process.

In vertical splitting, which corresponds to dissociation, there is a vertical defensive barrier within the ego. Threatening material is held in a dissociated compartment of the ego, where secondary process dominates the psychic functions. Thus, in the psychotherapy of DID, one can find out about events for which the host personality is amnesic simply by asking an alter personality. There is no need to explore "the unconscious." The alter personality has always remembered and no information has been repressed into the id. The two bodies of theory lead to radically different therapy procedures.

The scientific status of repression has no more relevance for the reliability and validity of dissociative disorders than it does for any other category in DSM-IV.

PROFESSIONAL SKEPTICISM ABOUT DISSOCIATIVE DISORDERS

Professional skepticism about dissociative disorders is often based on incorrectly equating dissociation with repression.[14–17] An example of a professional who does not diagnose DID is Helen Morrison,[18] a psychiatrist who interviewed about 80 serial killers before writing a book on the subject. Morrison states that none of the killers she interviewed had DID, even though one, John Gacy, described one of his alter personalities to her by name and function.

Gacy said to Dr. Morrison, "One body, two persons. The active person, John Gacy, has fifteen characters, not personalities, see? Fifteen different characters involved in one man. The sex drive, when it breaks in, it's two people, John Gacy and Jack Hanley... This guy Jack controls me. Eighteen hours of the day... He comes out. He comes out!... How the hell do I get him out? I don't know how to talk to him. I don't know how to bring him out" (p. 100).

While denying that Gacy had DID, Morrison testified at trial that, "There is a defense mechanism called splitting, and that's where the ego detaches from reality. For example, in Mr. Gacy, this is shown by his lack of memory for certain things." She then explains in her book, commenting on her testimony, that, "By 'certain things' I meant the killings themselves along with the recollection of portions of his own life" (p. 113).

Speaking generally of serial killers, Morrison states that, "Multiple murderers have a much deeper inner disorganization that is not really seen until they're in the middle of a crime or just as the crime is beginning. At that point, they're like Dr. Jekyll and Mr. Hyde. They fall apart and they come back together again" (p. 72). Elsewhere, she states that, "As we've seen, this is typical behavior for a serial killer. As if at the flip of a coin, their aspect, their external selves, change" (p. 215).

Dr. Morrison also had confirmatory collateral history about Gacy's childhood dissociation from his sister, Karen: "I remember that he once passed out at the top of the stairs and didn't remember when he came to. He was like someone who was drunk, but he wasn't drunk. Something in his voice was different. It was not *his* voice" (p. 88).

Dr. Morrison, John Gacy, and his sister, Karen, are all describing the same thing, which in DSM-IV is classified as dissociative identity disorder. The vocabulary varies depending who is describing the dissociation: Karen says "it's not his voice"; John Gacy says it's "Jack Hanley" who has "come out" but insists that Jack Hanley is a different "character" not a different "personality"; while Dr. Morrison says that a defense called splitting has resulted in a detachment of Gacy's ego from reality that in turn has resulted in amnesia for his crimes. She refers to the detached component of Gacy's ego as an "external aspect."

Dr. Morrison considers DID to be extremely rare, but she simultaneously describes the phenomenon of DID as being typical of serial killers. In a debate, she might adopt the position that she has never seen a serial killer with DID, but the differences between her descriptions of serial killers and my clinical descriptions of sex offenders are entirely semantic. The substance is identical.

I propose that this is generally true throughout the paraphilias: dissociative disorders including DID are common—but not recognized. The phenomenology is observed and described, but accounted for with different vocabulary: dissociation becomes splitting; alter personalities become, perhaps, behavioral states; amnesia becomes forgetting; dissociative voices become psychotic voices; disavowal of behavior based on genuine amnesia becomes lying, and so on.

The fear that a diagnosis of DID might result in a not guilty verdict for the host personality is easily put to rest for serial killers, and for sex offenders in general. There is never complete amnesia, and the host personality is as guilty as a separate person driving the getaway car. The host personality colludes with the offender personality, and carefully avoids detection and arrest. The host personality is a direct accomplice and is also consciously harboring a fugitive.

A DISSOCIATIVE STRUCTURAL MODEL OF THE PSYCHE

For dissociative disorders to be relevant to understanding sex offenders, several things must be true: it must be possible to diagnose dissociative disorders with good reliability and concurrent validity; the dissociative disorders cannot be rare; and, specifically, they cannot be rare among sex offenders. Additionally, in my view, a dissociative structural model of the psyche is required to make sense of the psychology of the sex offender, or at least of the subgroup of offenders to whom this model applies.

I propose that a structural dissociative model of the psyche is required to make clinical sense of a range of DSM-IV symptoms and disorders. The list of diagnoses includes DID and DDNOS, posttraumatic stress disorder (PTSD), somatoform disorders, borderline personality disorder (BPD), obsessive-compulsive disorder (OCD), some subtypes of schizophrenia, and impulse control disorders.

This is a structural model, not an etiological model. In principle, a dissociated executive self could arise from any number of causes, including faulty DNA, intrauterine infections, and psychological trauma. In practice, psychological trauma is the major etiological factor, but it is not required absolutely.

For whatever set of reasons, in DID, DDNOS, and related disorders in the spectrum covered by the model, the executive self, ego, or conscious mind is not an integrated structure. Instead, it is broken down into subcomponents or modules that have varying degrees of disconnection between them. There is a deficit in information flow between the modules, which can include components of memory, arousal, sensation, cognition, perception, movement, or any other function. The deficit, blockage, or dissociation can be partial or complete and the degree of dissociation can fluctuate over time.

I am using a variety of interchangeable terms here to emphasize that the model does not hinge on the semantics of any one school of psychology.

The self, in this model, is composed of a set of subsystems that lack the normal degree of fluidity, integration, and information exchange seen in a healthy psyche. Instead of one self, there is a collection of subselves. In DID, the various subselves are dissociated to an extreme degree, and they are personified and elaborated to an extreme degree. In DID, there are different "people" inside.

In DDNOS, there is the same psychological structure, but to a lesser degree. The degree of dissociation is not as extreme, the amnesia is less dense and less complex, there is more leakage across the system, the subselves are less invested in being separate, and the switches of executive control are less clear. Most people with full DID, in fact, function at the DDNOS-level much of the time and across many of their systems.

Typically, DID is a mixture of DDNOS-level function and DID-level function. Both categories, however, are in the dissociative taxon.

When a dissociated structure is in place, a number of phenomena can follow. If there is a full amnesia barrier between subselves, complete switching of executive control, and full personification of the subselves, then classical DID is present. However, even in a classical case of DID, most of the symptoms are caused by interactions between the subselves (the different "parts," "people," "alter personalities," "characters," or "external aspects," depending on one's vocabulary) that do not involve full switching, complete amnesia, or fully separate identities.

In the DID literature, the part-self in executive control most of the time is referred to as the *host personality*. The host personality is not "the real person," any more or less than any of the other parts. The "real person" is the sum of all the parts. Indeed, the current host personality may have been functioning as the host personality for only a few years, or there may be a group of identity states that share the host personality tasks.

Most of the interactions between the parts take the form of *intrusions* and *withdrawals*, rather than full switches of executive control. Let's say that Mary is the host, while Alice and Susan are other personalities in the system. Mary is devoid of feelings, recalls little childhood abuse, goes to work, and performs some domestic tasks. She does not nurture the children or have sex with "the husband." Alice is a frightened child who was sexually abused by her father. Alice has PTSD and likes to play with Mary's children. Susan is a promiscuous teenager who despises Mary's children. She is unfaithful to "Mary's husband" but has sex with him on demand.

Mary hears Susan yelling at Alice inside her head: she previously received a diagnosis of schizophrenia because of these auditory hallucinations. DSM-IV criteria state that schizophrenia can be diagnosed when the only symptom present is voices talking to each other or commenting on the person's actions. When Mary's husband makes sexual advances to her, Alice's PTSD is triggered and Mary experiences terror and then freezes, due to leakage from Alice. She hears Alice crying, then remembers nothing till the next morning, when her husband thanks her for the great sex the previous night.

Occasionally, Mary finds herself watching her body as if from above and outside it—she sees herself dialing an unknown phone number and then talking in a seductive voice to a man on the other end of the line who seems to know her and calls her Susan. Mary comes back into her body, apologizes for dialing the wrong number, and hangs up. These symptoms are intrusions into the executive self without switching.

As with the Schneiderian symptoms of schizophrenia, feelings, thoughts, or actions can be created, depending on what is intruding from another self-state. Withdrawal symptoms include amnesia, Schneiderian thought withdrawal, conversion paralyses, aphonia, and emotional numbness.

Many of the positive symptoms of schizophrenia could not occur without a dissociated psychological structure. It is not possible to hear ego-alien voices that are not under executive control unless those voices are arising from a dissociated sector of the psyche. Otherwise, they would be one's own thoughts or internal monologue, not auditory hallucinations. The more complex, interactive, and rich the voices, the larger and more elaborated the self-state from which they originate.

Conversely, the more rigid, unvaried, and rote voices arise from a smaller and less personified sector of psyche that is less easily engaged in psychotherapy.

Consider OCD: by definition, OCD involves the intrusion of ego-alien thoughts and impulses into the executive self. If there were no structural dissociation, such intrusions could not occur. There would be nowhere for them to intrude from. When the intruding content is an "impulse" then the diagnosis is an impulse control disorder, such as trichotillomania. In my view, compulsive hair-pulling should not be in a separate diagnostic category from compulsive hand-washing. Neither can occur unless there is a dissociated part-self from whom the impulse or compulsion arises.

Treatment techniques such as response prevention and thought stopping, and pharmacological strategies for OCD, involve reinforcing the dissociation and walling off the sector of psyche from which the obsessions and compulsions arise. An alternative strategy is psychotherapeutic integration of the dissociated part-self, so that it can no longer give rise to ego-alien intrusions.

Using similar logic, PTSD could be called *bipolar trauma disorder*. The "up" pole of the disorder consists of terror, autonomic hyperarousal, flashbacks, startle reactions, and other intrusions into the executive self. The "down" pole consists of an emptied-out withdrawal state in which there is numbing, avoidance, social withdrawal, and shut-down. The numbing phase represents successful dissociation and the active phase represents a failure of dissociation. Most people with PTSD oscillate back and forth between these two poles.

The same "bipolar" model could be applied to the positive and negative symptoms of schizophrenia. In a subset of persons with schizophrenia, the negative symptoms could be due to a dissociative shut-down and emptying out of the executive self. The negative symptoms, in a subgroup of individuals, could be related to failure of bonding and nurturance by the parents, and overt child neglect, compounded by institutionalization, social stigma, medication side effects and concurrent depression.

Intermittent explosive disorder represents a sudden, catastrophic intrusion of a rage state into the executive self. According to DSM-III,[19] episodes of intermittent explosive disorder are often accompanied by amnesia. The same analysis can be applied to somatoform disorders, which represent intrusions and withdrawals of a physiological state. Indeed, amnesia is a symptom of somatoform disorder and in ICD-10,[20] dissociative and conversion disorders belong to the same category. ICD-10 recognizes that dissociations can occur in sensation, physiological arousal, movement, and the five senses, whereas DSM-IV limits dissociation to memory, identity, and cognition.

The symptoms of BPD can also be accounted for within this structural dissociation model because all represent either intrusions into the executive self (impulsive behavior and mood instability), or withdrawals from the executive self (emptiness and boredom, loss of identity, or identity confusion).

This structural model does not imply that everyone with these various disorders "really" has DID. It is assumed that in most cases the dissociated part-selves are less personified, less differentiated, and less fully dissociated than they are in full DID. The dissociative structural model is not so much a theory as a logical argument: a wide range of intrusion and withdrawal symptoms cannot occur unless there is a disconnected, ego-alien sector of the psyche that inserts and withdraws the thoughts, impulses, feelings, memories, compulsions, voices, physiological sensations, motor and perceptual functions, and indeed any psychic function.

The symptoms are reported by the executive self, who is regarded as "the person," but the other dissociated part-selves can also be engaged in the therapeutic process. When they are integrated, both the intrusions and the withdrawals cease. An operationalized model of therapy can be applied to any person with a dissociated psychological structure, no matter what combination of comorbid symptoms and diagnoses is in place.

A COMPOSITE PROFILE OF A DISSOCIATIVE SEX OFFENDER

A composite case description of a sex offender with a dissociated psychological structure follows:

H.A. is a 42-year-old divorced man referred for specialty inpatient treatment by the courts as a condition of his sentencing for indecent exposure. He admits to sexually abusing his daughter, whom he has not seen for 6 years. He spends hundreds of dollars per week on adult female prostitutes, admits to committing two rapes as a teenager, and also cruises for adolescent male prostitutes on occasion. Several girlfriends have told him that they are ending their relationship with him because he is a sex addict.

Mr. A. used cocaine heavily from age 22 to 34 but has not used it since. He drank alcohol heavily from late adolescence till age 38. He has not abused any substances since. He meets criteria for major depressive episode, recurrent, currently active. He does not have a history of criminal behavior other than his paraphilias.

Mr. A. states that he wants to quit his sex addiction, but the urges become too overwhelming to suppress. He describes an inner battle to keep the urges down. When he has fought his "inner demons" for too long, he finally acquiesces, knowing that after he acts out, there will be a refractory period during which he experiences no urges or internal conflict.

Although Mr. A. does not describe any frank amnesia, he says that his memory of cruising for prostitutes is often "fuzzy" the next day, and he describes significant time distortion while cruising—4 or 5 hours can seem like 15 minutes. He describes experiencing some of his acting out from a depersonalized perspective, especially when he hires adolescent male prostitutes to penetrate him anally.

Mr. A. also masturbates compulsively in front of the mirror while dressed in women's underwear he has stolen by breaking into apartments. He says that he sometimes watches the masturbation from outside his body—during those occasions, the person in the mirror looks like a pre-pubertal girl. Sometimes he hears an angry, sarcastic, accusatory voice telling the girl in the mirror that she is a slut.

Mr. A. reports a history of childhood sexual abuse by his mother and his maternal grandfather. His mother used to dress him up in her clothes before forcing him to engage in mutual masturbation. He says that when he is receiving anal intercourse from an adolescent boy prostitute, he sometimes feels like a girl.

Mr. A. recognizes that his sexual addiction is similar to his alcohol and cocaine abuse, in that it helps him deny, suppress, and avoid his anger, grief, anxiety, and inner conflicts. He says that he is really a normal person, he just has these urges coming from inside that he can't control.

Mr. A. experiences a wide range of symptoms from many different sections of DSM-IV, including somatoform, borderline personality, posttraumatic stress, and impulse control disorders. All these symptoms have responded partially, at best, to trials of many different antidepressants and mood stabilizers.

According to the dissociative structural model, Mr. A.'s psyche is likely fragmented into a set of subidentities. When Mr. A. claims to be a "normal person," he is correct as far as his executive self is concerned. In the workplace he is high functioning and regarded as a normal person, because the structured environment and tasks allow him to keep his dissociative intrusions at bay. He acts out sexually during evenings and weekends, but not at work.

Based on the brief case history above, the subselves likely include a girl who was sexually abused by the mother and who has passive anal intercourse with male prostitutes; an angry, critical state identified with the mother; an executive self; and a heterosexual adolescent male who picks up female prostitutes. When the executive self claims that he is not a sex addict, this is not simply denial or lying: it is psychologically true of the executive self, but not true of the whole person. Treatment can go in one of two directions: suppression or integration of the disavowed part-selves. Integrative treatment necessarily includes containment, consequences for acting out, and limit setting and clear boundaries by the therapist. It is not permissive or indulgent. The ultimate goals of the two approaches, however, are radically different.

FUTURE RESEARCH

Considerable research effort would be required for the dissociative structural model of paraphilias to be generally accepted. First, many replications of the basic diagnostic findings are required: the size of the dissociative subgroup within sex offenders and addicts must be established across a range of samples and populations. The more extreme the offender, I predict, the greater the degree of trauma, dissociation, and comorbidity.

The second phase would consist of treatment outcome studies. An integrative therapy model would have to be tested against other approaches using standard outcome measures including symptom measures, recidivism rates, and disturbed arousal patterns.

SUMMARY

A dissociative structural model of the psyche can account for a wide range of symptoms across many DSM-IV categories, including sexual compulsions and addictions. The model leads to a distinct overall plan of treatment and a set of operationalized interventions aimed at integration of the self, rather than suppression of impulses. The model could be tested first in epidemiological studies and later in treatment outcome studies.

REFERENCES

1. Ellason JW, Ross CA. Childhood trauma and dissociation among male sex offenders. Sexual Addictions and Compulsivity 1999;6:105–10.
2. Ross CA. Dissociative identity disorder: diagnosis, clinical features, and treatment of multiple personality. 2nd edition. New York: John Wiley & Sons; 1997.
3. Ross CA. The trauma model: a solution to the problem of comorbidity in psychiatry. Richardson (TX): Manitou Communications; 2007.
4. Bernstein EM, Putnam FW. Development, reliability and validity of a dissociation scale. J Nerv Ment Dis 1986;174:727–35.
5. Steinberg M. Handbook for the assessment of dissociation: a clinical guide. Washington, DC: American Psychiatric Pres; 1995.
6. Dell PF. Dissociative phenomenology of dissociative identity disorder. J Nerv Ment Dis 2002;190:10–5.
7. Ross CA, Duffy CMM, Ellason JW. Prevalence, reliability and validity of dissociative disorders in an inpatient setting. J Trauma Dissociation 2002;3:7–17.
8. Pincus HA, Rush AJ, First MB, et al. Handbook of psychiatric measures. Washington, DC: American Psychiatric Association; 2000.
9. Cohen NJ, Eichenbaum H. Memory, amnesia, and the hippocampal system. Cambridge (MA): MIT Press; 1993.
10. Breuer J, Freud S. Studies on hysteria. New York: Pelican; 1986.

11. Masson JM. The complete letters of Sigmund Freud to Wilhelm Fleiss 1887–1904. Cambridge (MA): Belknap Press; 1985.

12. Freud S. Repression (1915). In: Rief P, editor. Freud: general psychological theory. New York: Touchstone Books; 1963. p. 104–15.

13. Hilgard ER. Divided consciousness: multiple controls in human thought and action. New York: John Wiley & Sons; 1977.

14. Merskey H. The manufacture of personalities. In: Cohn L, Berzoff J, Elin M, editors. Dissociative identity disorder: theoretical and treatment controversies. Northvale (NJ): Jason Aronson; 1995. p. 3–32.

15. Pope HG, Oliva PS, Hudson JI, et al. Attitudes towards DSM-IV dissociative disorders diagnoses among board-certified American psychiatrists. Am J Psychiatry 1999;165:321–3.

16. Piper A. Hoax and reality: the bizarre world of multiple personality disorder. Northvale (NJ): Jason Aronson; 1997.

17. Mai F. Psychiatrist's attitudes towards multiple personality disorder: a questionnaire survey. Can J Psychiatry 1995;40:154–7.

18. Morrison H. My life among serial killers: inside the minds of the world's most notorious murderers. New York: Avon Books; 2004.

19. American Psychiatric Association. Diagnostic and statistical manual of mental disorders. 3rd edition. Washington, DC: Author; 1980.

20. World Health Organization. ICD-10: the ICD-10 classification of mental and behavioral disorders. Clinical descriptions and diagnostic guidelines. Geneva (Switzerland): Author; 1992.

Basic Science and Neurobiological Research: Potential Relevance to Sexual Compulsivity

Fred S. Berlin, MD, PhD

KEYWORDS

- Sexual addiction • Sexual compulsivity
- Sexual drive • Paraphilias • Endorphins
- Opiate receptors

WHAT IS SEXUAL COMPULSIVITY?

Reportedly, the eminent neurologist Hughlings Jackson (1835–1911) once said that "the study of causes must first be preceded by the study of things caused." That is so, regardless of whether any given cause is predominately neurobiologic, psychological, or cultural in its origins. In this instance, before one can adequately address issues related to the science and neurobiology of sexual compulsivity, it is first necessary to have a clear operational definition of precisely what it is that constitutes a sexually compulsive act. In practical terms, successful neurobiologic research frequently has been enhanced when an accepted animal model of the phenomenon has been studied. Putting aside artificially induced sexual acts, however, acts that can occur in relationship either to stimulation or ablation of focalized brain neurons,[1] there has been no scientific consensus regarding a naturally occurring animal model of sexually compulsive behavior.

Further complicating matters, if one hopes to extrapolate the results of animal research to the human condition, it is necessary to factor into the equation not only the relevant distinctions between various species but also the role of culture. For instance, arguably engaging in multiple concurrent sexual relationships in a society that values monogamy might be seen as an example of sexual compulsivity. Such actions might not be viewed in that same way in a polygamous culture—a culture in which a married man with several wives might experience little need to resist having concurrent relationships.

By its nature, all sexual behavior is a driven—if not compulsive—act, an act that is energized by a powerful biologic appetite. Deciding not to give into sexual temptation

Department of Psychiatry and Behavioral Sciences, The John Hopkins University School of Medicine, Baltimore, MD, USA
E-mail address: fredsberlinmd@comcast.net

Psychiatr Clin N Am 31 (2008) 623–642
doi:10.1016/j.psc.2008.07.003
0193-953X/08/$ – see front matter © 2008 published by Elsevier Inc.

can represent much more of a challenge than deciding not to put on a particular pair of earrings, a special tie, or a favorite bracelet. Although we rarely pause to think about it, sexual desire is much more the product of biology than logic.

Sexual drive can vary in its intensity (quantitatively) and its orientation or aim (qualitatively).[2] If not unduly intense, an erotic drive whose aim repeatedly leads a man to be desirous of intimacy in a consensual fashion might not cause problems of a sexually compulsive nature. On the other hand, a drive whose aim repeatedly leads a man to be desirous of nonconsensual intimacy, as can occur in sexual sadism, might cause such problems. That could be so to the extent that a man with a sadistic sexual makeup experiences difficulty in resisting his particular sort of erotic cravings— resistance that might not even be necessary or relevant in the case of a man who has never experienced sadistic cravings in the first place.[3] A misdirected sexual drive can occur in paraphilic disorders such as sadism, necrophilia, or pedophilia.[4] In addition to its relationship to the intensity of sexual drive, sexual compulsivity also can be related to the direction in which that drive is aimed along with society's willingness—or lack thereof—to allow its expression.

When addressing the matter of sexual compulsivity, some researchers have spoken about sexual desire in its pure form (ie, lust). Others have hypothesized about pathologies thought to be associated with the desire to find a mate (eg, abnormalities of the so-called "mating" or "courtship" instincts). Still others have approached the issue more broadly, addressing affects such as loneliness and the need to feel intimacy and love.[5–7] Although not ordinarily eroticized, some have related the notion of sexual compulsivity to various forms of addiction or to other sorts of compulsions. Finally, proponents of the concept have been accused of attempting to excuse sin by relabeling it psychopathology. The argument is that sexual behaviors are indulged not for compulsive reasons but because they feel so good. The counter argument is that it is precisely because they feel so good that successful resistance can be so difficult. Given the complexities of defining and perhaps even agreeing about what constitutes the essence of sexual compulsivity, what—if anything—can be said about any associated neurobiology?

THE NEUROBIOLOGY OF FACTORS RELATED TO RESISTING SEXUAL URGES

Ordinarily, at least two opposing forces are at play when addressing the matter of sexual compulsivity. First, there is a drive that craves satiation that under circumstances not requiring resistance would likely be satisfied routinely. In the absence of any need to resist, we retire when sleepy, drink when thirsty, think more about food and eat when hungry, urinate when the bladder is full, and take a breath of air when in need of oxygen. Second, there is the impetus to resist. It is only by trying to resist the force of a biologic drive and discovering that we cannot do so consistently that concepts such as volitional impairment, addiction, or compulsion begin to take on any relevance.

All else being equal, arguably a brain-damaged, demented, depressed, or mentally retarded individual with poor coping skills might be more at the mercy of a strong sexual drive than would be a more gifted or intact person. A sober person may be more capable of resisting than would one who is intoxicated. Some may have a greater appreciation of the importance of resisting than others. A strong drive sometimes can color one's ability to perceive that importance objectively. The sociopathic individual, who lacks a sense of conscience and moral responsibility, might not be in a position to even discover whether he or she can resist successfully because often he or she may not make the effort to do so. A discussion of the neurobiologic correlates of the capacity, or willingness, to resist acting on troublesome or unacceptable sexual urges is beyond the scope of this article. This article does not explore the neurobiology of character, personality, or temperament or any associated comorbidities.

THE CONCEPT OF CHOICE

Regardless of character, the force of a strong drive—whether innate or acquired—sometimes can be sufficiently persistent so as to wear down, at least intermittently, the best of intentions, chosen resolve, and personal commitment. The notion that one can invariably successfully chose to indefinitely resist an intense urge is often simply incorrect. For example, because of the intense fear elicited when a gunman proclaims "your money or your life," there is little margin for choice. Similarly, there may be little margin for choice when it comes to certain biologically based imperatives. When resisting the urge to breath, urinate, or sleep, any such choice is inevitably bound to fail eventually. From the perspective of preservation of the species, satisfying sexual desire is also a biologic imperative. Without adequate treatment, when faced with powerful and perhaps even overpowering biologically based erotic cravings, the sexually compulsive individual also may be headed for failure. Contending that one should be able to resist successfully does not constitute proof that one is actually capable of consistently doing so. The degree of choice available to any given individual over time is not a constant.

Some researchers have suggested that masturbation can decrease the urge to act in a sexually improper manner. In some instances it can, at least for awhile. For some individuals, however, masturbation may whet sexual appetite in the long run rather than reduce it. Accessing sexually explicit imagery in order to masturbate may momentarily trigger a heightened sexual desire. On the other hand, one cannot permanently eliminate sexual desire by refraining from masturbation. The intensity of sexual desire is ordinarily cyclical. Once satiated, it heightens again over time. For many sexually compulsive individuals, a choice to permanently refrain from masturbating may not be possible. For sexually compulsive persons, the frequency of masturbation often may be more of a gauge of the intensity of sexual desire rather than an unencumbered choice.

Parents do not need to teach their children how to become heterosexual, bisexual, or homosexual in orientation. A heterosexual male does not need to be introduced to *Playboy* magazine to develop an erotic interest in women. Nor is it necessary that he recurrently "reinforce" that interest by looking at such images for that interest to be sustained. Conversely, refraining from viewing such imagery does not cause him to lose that interest. Whether because of genetics, imprinting, or other sorts of early life experiences, one discovers rather than chooses the qualitative orientation and the inherent quantitative intensity of one's sexual makeup. Once there, one ordinarily cannot chose to engage in acts or refrain from engaging in acts so as to significantly alter or eliminate that makeup. Throughout his early years, ordinarily a young man with a strong and exclusively heterosexual makeup is likely to remain a young man with a strong and exclusively heterosexual makeup. Given the premise that many aspects of sexual desire are about matters other than choice, what are those other factors?

TESTOSTERONE: ITS RELATIONSHIP TO THE INTENSITY OF SEXUAL DRIVE AND POSSIBLE LINK TO SEXUAL COMPULSIVITY

Because the concept of sexual compulsivity is so new, there is little, if any, knowledge about any associated neurobiology. The question becomes what can be learned from animal and other basic science research about broader issues of sexually motivated behavior and how—if at all—that knowledge can be applied to the issue at hand. An extensive body of relevant scientific data is available about biologic and neurobiologic factors that are associated with the sexual drive itself and with its intensity. Arguably, the concept of sexual compulsivity may be tied intimately to that intensity dimension. Much of the relevant research regarding that matter dates back to the period during which the hormone testosterone initially was identified. The chemical structure of testosterone is depicted in **Fig. 1**.

As documented in *Wikipedia*, testosterone's history has been interesting.[8] The association between testicular activity and circulating substances in the blood was first appreciated and studied in the early 1800s by Arnold Bethold. His work involved castration and testicular transplantation in fowl. Several decades later, in 1899, Harvard Professor Charles-Edward Brown-Sequard, then residing in Paris, published a study in a British medical journal, *The Lancet*, that reported on subcutaneous self-injection of an extract of dog and guinea pig testicles—work that subsequently was ridiculed by colleagues. Not until approximately 30 years later, when a professor of physiologic chemistry at the University of Chicago, Fred C. Koch, succeeded in accessing a large source of bovine testicles from the Chicago stock yards, did the next major advances begin to occur. In 1927, Koch and his student, Lemuel McGee, derived a mere 20 mg of an as yet unidentified substance from a supply of nearly 40 lb of bull testicles. When administered to castrated roosters, pigs, and rats, the substance "remasculinized" the animals. Approximately 12 years later, in 1939, two researchers, Adolf Butenandt and Leopold Ruzicka, who worked out the structure of that previously unidentified substance (testosterone) and a preliminary understanding of its synthesis through a series of steps from cholesterol, shared the Nobel Prize in chemistry.

From a biologic perspective, testosterone is a remarkable hormone. As a consequence of possessing a Y chromosome, the male fetus develops functional testes before birth, which in turn produce testosterone. That testosterone then causes

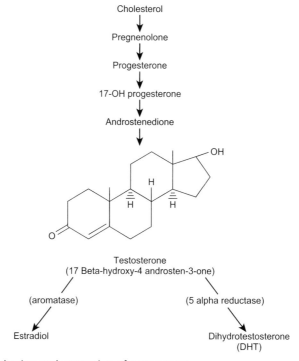

Cholesterol
↓
Pregnenolone
↓
Progesterone
↓
17-OH progesterone
↓
Androstenedione
↓

Testosterone
(17 Beta-hydroxy-4 androsten-3-one)

(aromatase)   (5 alpha reductase)

Estradiol   Dihydrotestosterone
                               (DHT)

Fig. 1. The production and conversion of testosterone.

what would otherwise have become the female labia to transform into the male scrotal sac, and it causes the clitoris to transform into a penis.[9] Testosterone is why a male infant even looks like a male at birth. Exposure of the fetus to testosterone also "masculinizes" the male brain; for example, preventing the subsequent cyclical surge of gonadotropic pituitary hormones that is associated with monthly menstruation in women. It also seems to alter the developing cerebral cortex in such a fashion that mathematical skills are associated with somewhat different areas of the brain in men as opposed to women. At the time of puberty, boys experience a marked surge in testosterone production, which is associated with a deepening of the male voice, the development of a male bodily habitus, the growth of facial hair, and a markedly heightened increase in sexual drive.[10]

Testosterone and other related androgenic hormones also seem to be associated with the intensity of sexual desire in women. That conclusion is supported by at least two lines of human research. For instance, in one double-blind study, women who complained of a low level of sexual desire experienced a heightened libido after administration of low doses of testosterone but not after administration of a placebo.[11] In a somewhat different but conceptually related study, researchers kept track of when a group of women most often initiated sexual activity in contrast to being the recipient of their partners' advances.[12] The women were most likely to initiate sexual activity at a time during their monthly cycle when testosterone-related hormones were at their peak. Functional MRI has documented neurobiologic changes within the brains of women that are believed to be important to sexual arousal and would seem to be in synchrony with androgenic hormonal variances in their menstrual cycles.[13]

A fair amount is known from a neurobiologic perspective about how testosterone exerts its effects within the brain. For example, when a male animal is castrated (ie, when its testes are removed), there is ordinarily a subsequent marked reduction in sexually motivated behavior. Although the administration of testosterone can reverse that outcome, it is not able to do so if its conversion in the brain to estradiol is enzymatically blocked.[14] This fact suggests that it is estradiol, to which testosterone is converted in the brain, that functions as the active neurotransmitter with respect to energizing and intensifying sexual drive. Although the major source of testosterone production in males is a peripheral organ (ie, the testes), it is only because of that hormone's capacity to exert a central effect upon the brain that associated behavioral changes in sexual activity are likely to occur. Studies performed with men who have been castrated for various medical reasons and whose brains are exposed to less testosterone have documented a subjective motivational change (ie, a decreased subjective interest in sex).

Although most of the testosterone that is produced in males emanates from the testes, its adequate production greatly depends on neurobiologic activity in at least two areas of the brain: the hypothalamus and the pituitary gland.[15] Testosterone is also synthesized in smaller quantities in women by the thecal cells of the ovaries and by the placenta. It is produced in the zona reticularis of the adrenal gland in both sexes. Various aspects of these relationships are depicted schematically in **Fig. 2**.

Nature has provided a wide margin with respect to the levels of testosterone that are required in order to sustain sexual motivation and behavior. For example, with the possible exception of certain chromosomal conditions (eg, Klinefelter's syndrome) in a young, healthy adult man between the ages of 18 and 35, adequate sexual interest and capacity often can be maintained by testosterone levels varying anywhere between 275 and 875 ng of testosterone per 100 dL of blood.[16] On the other hand, levels of testosterone significantly below 275 ng/100 dL (eg, <100 ng/100 dL) are almost always associated with a low level of sexual motivation and behavior. It is

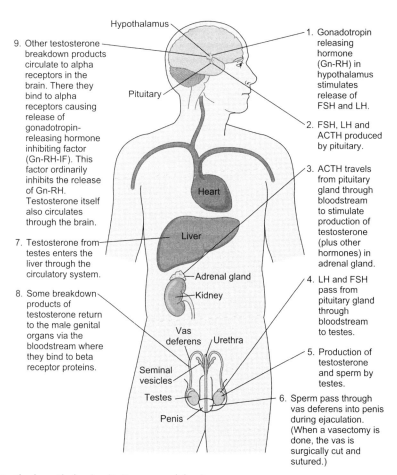

9. Other testosterone breakdown products circulate to alpha receptors in the brain. There they bind to alpha receptors causing release of gonadotropin-releasing hormone inhibiting factor (Gn-RH-IF). This factor ordinarily inhibits the release of Gn-RH. Testosterone itself also circulates through the brain.

7. Testosterone from testes enters the liver through the circulatory system.

8. Some breakdown products of testosterone return to the male genital organs via the bloodstream where they bind to beta receptor proteins.

Hypothalamus
Pituitary
Heart
Liver
Adrenal gland
Kidney
Vas deferens   Urethra
Seminal vesicles
Testes
Penis

1. Gonadotropin releasing hormone (Gn-RH) in hypothalamus stimulates release of FSH and LH.

2. FSH, LH and ACTH produced by pituitary.

3. ACTH travels from pituitary gland through bloodstream to stimulate production of testosterone (plus other hormones) in adrenal gland.

4. LH and FSH pass from pituitary gland through bloodstream to testes.

5. Production of testosterone and sperm by testes.

6. Sperm pass through vas deferens into penis during ejaculation. (When a vasectomy is done, the vas is surgically cut and sutured.)

Fig. 2. The hypothalamic-pituitary-gonadal axis.

not clear to what extent a pathologically elevated level of testosterone may be associated with a heightened sexual drive, although such a relationship would seem likely.

TREATMENT IMPLICATIONS

Because of testosterone's relationship to the intensity of sexual drive, as discussed elsewhere in this text, antiandrogens (medications capable of lowering testosterone) have been used as a means of facilitating appropriate sexual self-control in patients with a paraphilic disorder.[17–19] From a clinical perspective, it should be easier for a patient in treatment to resist satisfying his or her sexual appetite when the intensity of that appetite has been reduced significantly. By decreasing the intensity of sexual desire, sex drive–lowering medications often can heighten an individual's capacity to choose not to act. When testosterone-lowering methods have been used among sexual offenders, recidivism rates in general have been remarkably low.[20–22] That finding seems to suggest that lowering testosterone in persons who have shown evidence of sexual compulsivity, whether illegal or not, may constitute a viable treatment option.

It is important to emphasize that testosterone, although of great significance, is by no means the only biologic agent crucial to sustaining the intensity of sexual drive. Estradiol, a testosterone derivative, may function as a key neurotransmitter with respect to that issue. Given the fact that some researchers have equated the terms "sexual compulsivity" and "sexual addiction," opiates produced internally in the brain (ie, endorphins) also may play a significant role in sustaining—and perhaps even enhancing—erotic interests. That knowledge may not have any clear treatment applications currently, although it is conceivable that medications capable of lowering the craving for opiates eventually may turn out to be useful in treating sexual compulsivity.

Some researchers have correctly pointed out that the release of various other neurotransmitters besides estradiol and internally produced opiates may be relevant.[23-28] For example, some researchers have emphasized the possible relationship between sexual drive and the neurotransmitter serotonin.[29] It has been suggested that antidepressant medications such as fluoxetine (Prozac) and paroxetine (Paxil), both of which are selective serotonin reuptake inhibitors, might be helpful in reducing sexual compulsivity. Such drugs block the reuptake of serotonin into certain cells within the brain. For unclear reasons, however, although Prozac and Paxil block serotonin reuptake, Prozac is more likely to inhibit libido than Paxil. The use of any of the selective serotonin reuptake inhibitors for such a purpose is based on a much less compelling body of scientific knowledge than is the case for medications that lower testosterone, such as leuprolide (Depo-Lupron). Put simply, when prescribed in adequate dosages, testosterone-lowering medications far more reliably and consistently produce a marked decrease in sexual drive than other classes of drugs, including selective serotonin reuptake inhibitors. When prescribing any medication intended to lower sexual drive, the potential risks and benefits involved must be considered, along with other treatment options.

THE NEUROBIOLOGY OF QUALITATIVE DIFFERENCES IN SEXUAL MAKEUP

A diverse spectrum exists with respect to qualitative differences in sexual makeup among human beings.[30] For example, whereas most persons would feel disgusted about the thought of having sex with an animal, others clearly become aroused by such thoughts. Although most men would not even consider exposing themselves in public, some must struggle daily to prevent themselves from doing so.[31] Although some individuals (heterosexuals) have little or no interest in having sex with a member of the same gender, others (homosexuals) experience little or no erotic attraction to members of the opposite gender. Historically, it has been illegal in most countries for homosexual individuals to engage in intimate relationships with one another. Many persons were either unwilling, or unable, to refrain from doing so, however, and might have been viewed as sexually compulsive, although the term itself was not yet in vogue, in large part because of the qualitative nature of their sexual makeup.

Currently, despite a large volume of relevant research, there is little consensus within the scientific-medical community regarding specific neurobiologic processes that may be correlated with qualitative differences in sexual makeup.[32] Little is known about neurobiologic factors that may be correlated with sexual compulsivity, at least if the assumption is made (correctly or incorrectly) that in most instances any such neurobiology is related to something more than the intensity dimension of sexual drive.

Pedophilia is a psychiatric disorder in which the sexual drive is misdirected toward prepubescent children.[33-35] For good reasons, persons who have pedophilia need to resist succumbing to the temptation of becoming involved sexually with a child. Many persons afflicted with that disorder might rightfully be viewed as sexually compulsive, to the extent that they experience significant difficulties in resisting their pedophilic cravings. Although lowering the intensity of their pedophilic drives may make it easier to resist, ultimately being able to alter that sexual orientation neurobiologically would likely be of greater benefit. Currently, it is possible to reduce the intensity of sexual drive pharmacologically, largely because of an appreciation of the neurobiologic effects of lowering testosterone. With our current knowledge, clinicians are still far removed from the possibility of producing a qualitative alteration in sexual makeup via neurobiologic interventions, although some have claimed that stereotactic neuro-surgery may possess such potential.[36,37]

It is conceivable—and perhaps even probable—that in the future the neurobiologic processes that are likely correlated with qualitative differences in sexual makeup will be elucidated. Currently, there are some preliminary clues, although much more research and further replication are essential. To cite one example, when a group of seven men diagnosed with pedophilia were intravenously infused with a 100-μg dose of luteinizing hormone–releasing hormone, each responded with a significantly elevated release of luteinizing hormone from the brain into the blood stream, in comparison with controls.[38] That finding, although preliminary, seems to suggest the presence of some sort of atypical neurobiologic activity in the brains of men who were diagnosed with pedophilia.

Other research supports such a conclusion.[39–41] In one particularly unusual case, a 40-year-old man developed pedophilia de novo along with an inability to inhibit his sexual urges in association with the growth of a right orbitofrontal tumor.[42] His behavioral symptoms resolved fully after tumor resection. In a recent study that used MRI, researchers found decreased gray matter volumes within specific brain regions in 18 patients who had pedophilia, in comparison with heterosexual and homosexual control subjects.[43] The researchers reported that the differences found within the brains of patients who had pedophilia were similar to differences often detectable in persons who have obsessive-compulsive disorders.

ANIMAL AND OTHER BASIC SCIENCE RESEARCH: ITS POTENTIAL RELEVANCE TO AN UNDERSTANDING OF SEXUAL AND SEXUALLY COMPULSIVE BEHAVIORS IN HUMANS

Much research has been conducted with animals related to issues such as courtship, mating rituals, and sexual behavior in general.[44–50] Often the findings reported have been species specific; for example, gerbils are generally monogamous, whereas most other animals are not. Monogamous behaviors in animals have been linked to the activity of the neurotransmitter dopamine, especially with respect to its associated corticolimbic circuitry.[51] In most animal species, known biologic factors contribute significantly to sexual behavior, which can be witnessed by the fact that female dogs become sexually responsive to male dogs only while in heat (estrus). At such times, in response to the odor of chemical substances emitted from the female dogs, the male dogs become much more assertive sexually.

The instinctual aspects of sexual behavior in various animal species have been well documented and detailed.[52] For example, in the case of the stickleback fish, specific sequential configurations of visual stimuli can elicit (or "release") specific sexual responses.[53] Spiders and blow flies also respond to specific configurations of visual stimuli in a sexual way.[54] Male Siamese fighting fish are programmed genetically to respond aggressively to the sight of another male and sexually to the sight of a female. In some cases, animals are programmed genetically to respond sexually to sounds rather than vision. The sound of the wing beat of female crickets and mosquitoes is the stimulus that attracts males.[55] Even when instinctually based, however, the

In humans, as in animals, certain aspects of erotic functioning and certain differences in the brain between males and females seem to depend on exposure to various "sex hormones" during specific phases of embryonic development.[14,65–69] For example, females who were exposed prenatally to high doses of androgens tend to show patterns of psychosexual development as adults that are more typically seen in males.[70,71] Prenatal exposure to progesterone may have a "feminizing" effect.[72,73] Exposing a male human fetus to medications that contain estrogen may lead to patterns of adult psychosexual behaviors that are more commonly seen in women.[74,75]

"Hypersexuality" can occur in humans as a consequence of damage to various neuroanatomic structures. In one reported case, an adult male began to utter sexual obscenities and engage in exhibitionism and public masturbation after a thalamic infarct (a stroke).[76] None of these behaviors was present before his stroke. "Hypersexuality" (and pathologic gambling) has been reported as a rare side effect of the medication pramipexole dihydrochloride (Mirapex), a dopamine agonist, which is used to treat Parkinson's disease and restless leg syndrome.[77] Sexual disinhibition and even the de novo development of a paraphilic disorder have been reported as long-term sequelae of traumatic brain injury.[78] Patients who have Alzheimer's disease sometimes become either "hypersexual" or sexually disinhibited as their dementia progresses. In time, a better understanding of the multitude of factors that can contribute to sexual behavior in general—in animals and in humans—will lead to an enhanced appreciation of sexual compulsivity and its associated neurobiologic correlates.

FUTURE DIRECTIONS: BRAIN IMAGING AND THE BRAIN-MIND RELATIONSHIP

Studying animal sexuality has its obvious limitations if one is interested in extrapolating the results of any such research to human phenomenology (ie, mental experience) and behavior. Historically, the ability to search for any neurobiologic correlates of sexual behavior and experience, even in human research, has been limited significantly. Virtually no noninvasive techniques were available that would allow one to successfully correlate detectable neurobiologic changes in the brain with changes in subjective sexual experience in the mind. Philosophers have pondered for centuries the relationship between the brain as a physically functioning biologic organ and the mind as subjective experience. With the advent of certain newer forms of brain imaging, the ability to study that brain–mind relationship seems to be enhanced significantly. It may be possible to correlate subjective sexual feelings and behavior with regional brain metabolism and with specific sorts of focal neurochemical synaptic transmissions that take place within the human brain.

Historically, CT represented a significant step beyond traditional radiographs. For the most part, traditional radiographs were only able to reveal a flat two-dimensional image of solid structures, such as bone and other densities. The CT scan could go beyond that by producing three-dimensional images of the anatomic structure of softer tissues (eg, the structure of important organs such as the kidney, liver, and brain). CT is not capable of detecting and visualizing metabolic or specific chemical changes within such organs, however. A more advanced imaging technique, positron emission tomography (PET), is capable of doing so when performed on the human brain.[79–81]

PET scanning can be carried out by injecting a small bolus of radioactive labeled material known as a ligand into a peripheral vein, usually in the arm. The material, safe to humans because of its low dose of radiation, circulates through the blood stream and passes through every organ in the body, including the brain. Two types of organic substances important to brain functioning can be radioactively labeled or neurobiologic correlates of the observed sexual behaviors are often either only poorly understood or not understood at all.

In many species of birds, only the male sings. If a female zebra finch is administered estradiol as an embryo and androgen hormones as an adult, she sings a male courtship song, even without having heard it previously.[56] She also displays typical male mating behavior. Like normal males (but unlike normal females), she has an increased number of cells in the nucleus robustus archistratialis and other brain regions.

"Mounting" is a behavior that can be observed in rats. It involves placing the forepaws on the back of another while posturing the body in a fashion conducive to intercourse. Normally, only male rats do so; however, female rats that have been given testosterone at a specific time in utero subsequently manifest that behavior as adults.[57] Male rats do not normally build nests or care for their young, but they build nests and show other kinds of "maternal behavior" if electrical stimulation is applied to certain brain areas.[58]

Some animals have an innate predisposition to follow—and become psychologically attached to—the first object that they see moving in front of them during a "critical time period" in early life. Attractions acquired in this fashion are said to be "imprinted."[59] Researchers have described young ducks that became so imprinted toward a human being who replaced their mothers during that critical time period that they tried to feed him live worms—a drive apparently so strong that they tried to force them into his ears if he closed his mouth. Early life imprinting can influence the nature of an adult animal's subsequent sexual attractions. As is the case with animals, some aspects of human sexual behavior also seem to be biologically programmed, although a full understanding of related neurobiologic factors is lacking.[60–63] In humans, young adults are ordinarily perceived as erotically more attractive than elderly (or very young) persons, which makes sense in terms of nature's interest in procreation. Conceivably, such perceptions may be a function of biologically programmed brain circuitry.

A man does not have to be taught how to "thrust" when initially engaging in intercourse with a woman. Nor does he need to be taught how to achieve an erection. Instead, at some time in his life, because he has been biologically programmed to do so, he begins to have erections in response to specific sorts of tactile, olfactory, visual, or mental stimuli. Although some aspects of that response may be learned, its occurrence in the first place is unlearned.

A significant body of knowledge exists regarding the molecular, cellular, vascular, and peripheral neurologic mechanisms involved in achieving and sustaining a erection in human males. That knowledge has led to the development of performance-enhancing medications, such as sildenafil citrate (Viagra).[64] The physiologic mechanism of an erection involves the release of nitric oxide into the corpus cavernosum of the penis during sexual stimulation. That nitric oxide then activates a specific enzyme (guanylate cyclase), which leads to increased levels of cyclic guanosine monophosphate (cGMP). Increased levels of cGMP then produce smooth muscle relaxation and the inflow of blood, which result in an erection.

By inhibiting another enzyme (PDES), which is responsible for the degradation cGMP, sildenafil citrate allows it to accumulate, which consequently sustains smooth muscle relaxation, engorgement with blood, and the erection. Because of its direct effects on the penis, sildenafil citrate is capable of enhancing genital performance when a male becomes sexually aroused mentally. It cannot directly alter the intensity of sexual motivation, however, which depends largely on central neurobiologic activity in the brain itself. Although it does not act centrally in the brain, sildenafil citrate can affect receptor cells in the retina of the eye, which, in rare instances, can lead to visual impairment "tagged" chemically: (1) glucose and oxygen, both of which act as a source of energy to the brain, and (2) neurotransmitter substances, such as hormones (eg, estradiol), and opiates. As a radioactively labeled ligand such as glucose circulates through the brain, it becomes concentrated in particular regions if those regions are more active metabolically and require more glucose as a source of energy (and more blood). As a labeled neurotransmitter (eg, an opiate) circulates, it passes through and leaves brain regions that do not have opiate receptors and is taken up in areas of the brain that do. This is analogous to the way in which metal particles circulating by magnets pass by adjacent wood but stick to the magnets, which act as "receptors" that receive and hold them.

Once a radioactive labeled ligand has reached the brain, a computer connected to a Geiger counter–type device (or "scanner") placed around the head counts the number of radioactive particles (positrons) emitted per unit of time from specific anatomic sites. Because the scanner surrounds the head in a manner that enables "triangulation," a three-dimensional determination can be made of the precise source and depth of each emission. In turn, the integrated computer produces a series of viewable images based on those emissions. What is seen on each image is analogous to what would be seen if a cross-section of the brain were obtained by transecting it. The added advantage is that a record of the neurobiologic processes themselves also can be observed. Each image reflects the biologic processes that occurred at the time that the radioactivity was concentrated at the sites depicted. When a source of chemical energy, such as glucose, is radioactively labeled and injected, the images (or tomograms) produced reflect regional metabolic activities in the brain. When a neurotransmitter, such as an opiate, is radioactively labeled and injected, the images reflect focal neurosynaptic activities (as opposed to regional metabolism). This process is depicted in **Fig. 3**.

The phenomenon of human sexual arousal seems to be an excellent candidate for study by means of PET scanning. It can be produced mentally, it is experienced subjectively, it is correlated in the male with a readily observable physiologic change, it is sustainable over time, and as a biologic drive, it is related to factors of a neuroanatomic and hormonal nature. Detecting changes in the brain associated with sexual arousal can be important for several reasons. From a basic science standpoint, many intriguing questions can be posed.[82–84] For example, are the neurobiologic changes that occur in the brain during erotic arousal the same in men and women?[85] A study relevant to that question, which used functional MRI, documented the fact that the amygdala and the hypothalamus are more strongly activated in heterosexual men when viewing sexually arousing stimuli than in heterosexual women.[86] How would the brain respond to such inputs in persons who have pedophilia or in persons with a homosexual makeup? What effects are produced by other forms of sensory input such as tactile or olfactory? What changes are associated with arousal versus orgasm?[13] PET scanning has been used to document increased regional metabolic activity in a specific brain region (ie, the mesodiencephalic transitional area) during human male orgasm and ejaculation.[87] What changes are associated with sexually compulsive behavior and its subsequent treatment? In time, research may assist in further addressing these issues.

THE PURPOSE OF OPIATES AND OPIATE RECEPTORS WITHIN THE HUMAN BRAIN: ARE THEY RELATED TO SEXUAL COMPULSIVITY?

In 1974, before any knowledge that the brain produces its own opiates, two distinguished researchers, Saul Snyder and Candace Pert, made the discovery of

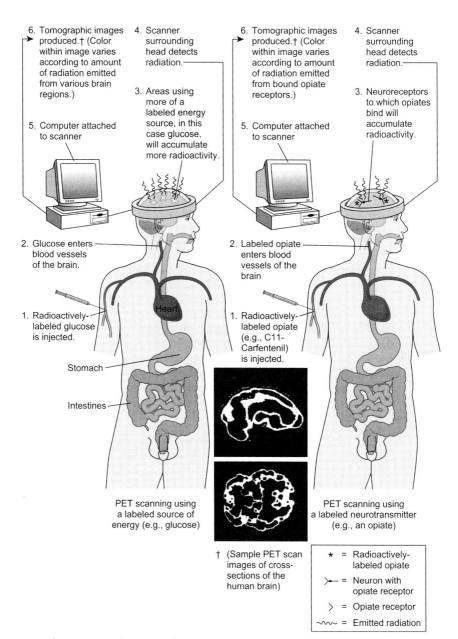

Fig. 3. The PET scanning procedure using either a radioactive labeled energy source (eg, glucose) or a radioactive labeled neurotransmitter (eg, an opiate).

neuroreceptors within the human brain to which opiates bind.[88] Initially that discovery seemed somewhat perplexing, because presumably those receptors, which are present in all human brains, were not there to bind to exogenously administered substances. Relatively few persons are ever exposed to either prescribed or illicit opiates during their lifetime. That matter became much less of a mystery, however, with the later discovery that the brain does manufacture its own internally produced opiates—substances known as endorphins.

Some researchers have observed that behaviors associated with sexual compulsivity sometimes can seem to be addictive in their nature. Is it possible that one of the many things that occurs within the human brain during sexual arousal is a release of endogenously produced opiates? If so, do some individuals (eg, persons who seem to be "sexually addicted") produce more such opiates than others? Do such persons have opiate receptors that are more sensitive than others? From an evolutionary perspective, it would be important to the survival of the species that sexual behavior be maintained. Perhaps the production and release of internally produced opiates in the brain during sexual activity might be one way of ensuring such maintenance. A fair amount of circumstantial evidence from basic science research already suggests that opiates may serve several functions within the brain, including playing an important role with respect to sexually motivated behaviors.[89–94] Before any of these matters can be addressed adequately, however, it is important to document the actual release of such opiates during sexual arousal within the human brain.

THE RELEASE OF INTERNALLY PRODUCED OPIATES IN THE HUMAN BRAIN DURING SEXUAL AROUSAL AS DOCUMENTED BY PET SCANNING

One way of determining whether internally produced opiates are actually being released by the brain during sexual arousal is through a two-stage study, with each investigational participant serving as his or her own control. This study already has been conducted. Within the first stage of that investigation, during which time study participants were not sexually aroused, a radioactive labeled mild opiate ligand with a short half-life (C11-carfentanil) was injected. It traveled through the blood stream to the brain, where some of it was bound by mu (but not by kappa) opiate receptors.

With the aid of an integrated computer, the Geiger counter–type device (the PET scanner) surrounding each participant's head was able to facilitate the production of pictures, or images, that varied in color according to the amount of radioactivity taken up by opiate receptors in various brain regions. The calcarine cortex, an area essentially devoid of opiate receptors, was used for control purposes to detect baseline levels of radiation within the brain caused by any labeled carfentanil that remained transitorily present, although unbound. Binding was deemed to have taken place at any given site only when the frequency of radioactive emissions from that site exceeded baseline levels.

During the second (or cross-over) stage of that study, the participants, who were all male hospitalized inpatients diagnosed with pedophilia at The Johns Hopkins Sexual Disorders Clinic in Baltimore, were asked to use mental imagery to become aroused. Arousal was confirmed by the presence of an erection. Radioactively labeled C-11 carfentinel was injected, and the PET scanning procedure was repeated. Researchers hypothesized that if internally produced opiates were being manufactured and released in the brain during sexual arousal and were binding to the brain's opiate receptors, less of the radioactive labeled carfentanil would be able to bind to those already occupied receptors than was case during the earlier nonaroused investigational session. If that was the case, the images obtained by PET scanning during the sexually aroused state should have shown less radioactivity emanating from those opiate receptors than was the case during the earlier nonaroused session. This process is depicted schematically in **Fig. 4**.

That study, which was supported in part by a research grant from the Guggenheim Foundation, provided evidence in seven of eight investigational participants of

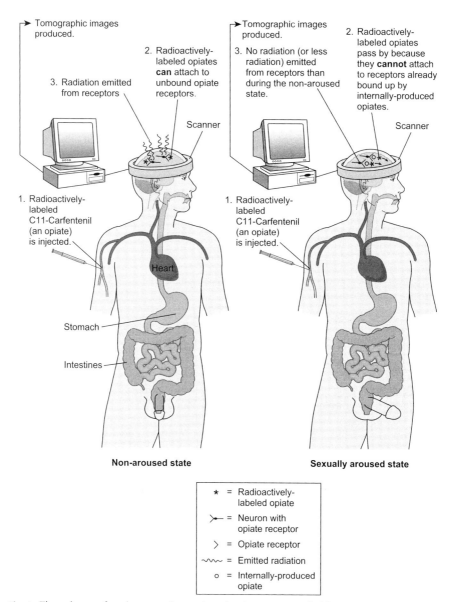

Fig. 4. The release of endogenously produced opiates as revealed by PET scanning.

a statistically significant release of internally produced opiates during sexual arousal in three brain regions.[95] Those three regions were the cingulate, the temporal cortex, and the frontal cortex. Significant opiate release was not observed in the caudate, the amygala, the thalamus, or the parietal cortex during sexual arousal, although all four of those regions, like the other three, contain high concentrations of opiate receptors. That research also documented a heightened synchronicity of opiate activity within the brain over time during sexual arousal. Four men who were unable to achieve erotic arousal within the study protocol showed no evidence of a heightened release of internally produced opiates when the results of their two PET scans were compared. Although this type of research requires additional replication and follow-up, it does demonstrate an investigational method that may help to further elucidate addictive-like neurobiologic changes within the brain possibly related to sexual compulsivity.

SUMMARY

A unique challenge posed by advancing scientific knowledge about the biology of human behavior is how to integrate that understanding with the desire to hold our-selves—and one another—morally accountable. As human beings, we are something more than just passive agents whose behavior is the sum product of biologic deter-minism. Because of the existence of the mind, we are also active agents with the capacity to influence, at least to some extent, our own destinies. Behavior may be determined, but it is not predetermined. We are one of its determinants. Misconduct by a person of sound mind should not be attributed improperly to brain pathology. On the other hand, suffering, legitimate mental disorder, and associated impairments should not be trivialized.

Historically, persons who once were labeled "lazy" are often more appropriately understood by modern standards as clinically depressed. Frequently they are more in need of pharmacologic treatments that alter brain chemistry than "a kick in the be-hind." Gluttony, one of the original cardinal sins, is often more properly understood as morbid obesity, a condition that deserves appropriate medical care. Persons who have alcoholism, once judged morally as "bums in the gutter," are more frequently referred to treatment facilities, such as The Betty Ford Clinic.

One should not approach the issue of human sexual behavior without at least some appreciation of moral values and scientific research. Although clearly some persons choose to act in a sexually selfish and self-indulgent fashion with wanton disregard, others seem to be more genuinely burdened and struggle to integrate their sexual desires into an otherwise healthy and fully responsible lifestyle. When a person, whether male or female, seems to be so driven that it becomes difficult to master erotic desires and he or she experiences difficulty serving his or her own best long-term interests, the concept of sexual compulsivity seems to be relevant. Ultimately, a better understanding of any associated neuropathologies may help to facilitate future treatments and public acceptance. The possibility exists, at least in some instances, that a sexually compulsive individual is less an example of a bad person deserving of punishment than a "broken mind" in need of repair. In time, increased knowledge about the precise workings of the brain in reciprocally initiating and sus-taining the sexual interests of the mind may facilitate a much clearer appreciation of the issues at hand.

ACKNOWLEDGMENTS

The author gratefully acknowledges the invaluable assistance of the following individuals: Denise G. Sawyer, Mary Anne Manner, Madenney Carlisle, Daniel J. Marshall, Adam Hoffberg, and Erica Sarr.

REFERENCES

1. Malsbury CW. Facilitation of male rat copulatory behavior by electrical stimulation of the medial preotic area. Physiol Behav 1971;7:797–805.
2. Berlin FS, Krout E. Pedophilia: diagnostic concepts, treatment and ethical consid-erations. Am J Forensic Psychiatry 1986;7(1):13–30.

3. Berlin FS. Criminal or patient? Culturefront 1998;5(2):71–5.
4. American Psychiatric Association. Diagnostic and statistical manual of mental disorders. 4th edition. [text revision]. Washington, DC: American Psychiatric Association; 2000. p. 566–76.
5. Carnes P. Sexual addiction. Minneapolis (MN): Compcare Publications; 1983.
6. Money J. Love and love sickness. Baltimore (MD): The Johns Hopkins University Press; 1981.
7. Kinsey AC, Pomeroy WB, Martin CE. Sexual behavior in the human male. Philadelphia: Saunders; 1948.
8. Available at: www.wikipedia.org. Accessed July 22, 2007.
9. Langmen J. Medical embriology. Baltimore (MD): Williams and Wilkins; 1969.
10. Berlin FS. Sex offenders: a biomedical perspective and a status report on biomedical treatment. In: Greer JB, Stuart IR, editors. The sexual aggressor: current perspectives on treatment II. New York: Van Nostrand Reinhold Co.; 1980. p. 82–123.
11. Carney A, Banacroft J, Mathews A. A combination of hormonal and psychological treatment for female sexual unresponsiveness: a comparative study. Br J Psychiatry 1978;132:339–46.
12. Adams DB, Gold AR, Burt AD. Raise in female initiated sexual activity at ovulation and its suppression by oral contraceptives. N Engl J Med 1980;299:1145–50.
13. Goldstein JM, Jerram M, Poldrack R, et al. Hormonal cycle modulates arousal circuitry in women using functional magnetic resonance imaging. J Neurosci 2005; 25(40):9309–16.
14. McEwen BS. Neural gonadal steroid actions. Science 1981;211:1303–11.
15. Whalen RE. Brain mechanisms controlling sexual behavior. In: Beach FA, editor. Human sexuality in four perspectives. Baltimore (MD): Johns Hopkins University Press; 1976. p. 311–20.
16. Berlin FS, Schaerf FW. Laboratory assessment of the paraphilias and their treatment with antiandrogenic medication. In: Hall RC, Beresford TP, editors. Handbook of psychiatric diagnostic procedures. New York: Spectrum Publications Inc.; 1985. p. 273–305.
17. Rosler A, Witztum E. Treatment of men with paraphilia with a long-acting analogue of gonadotropin releasing hormone. N Engl J Med 1998;338:416–22.
18. Bradford JM. Organic treatment for the male offender. Behav Sci Law 1985;3: 355–75.
19. Berlin FS, Meinecke CF. Treatment of sex offenders with antiandrogenic medication: conceptualization, review of treatment modulates and preliminary findings. Am J Psychiatry 1981;138:601–7.
20. Berlin FS. Commentary: the impact of surgical castration on sexual recidivism risk among civilly committed sexual offenders. J Am Acad Psychiatry Law 2005;33(1): 37–41.
21. Freund K. Therapeutic sex drive reduction. Acta Psychiatr Scand 1980; 287(Suppl):5–38.
22. Weinberger LE, Sreemivasan S, Garrick T, et al. The impact of surgical castration on sexual recidivism risk among sexually violent predatory offenders. J Am Acad Psychiatry Law 2005;33(1):16–36.
23. Kafka MP. A monoamine hypothesis for the pathophysiology of paraphilic disorders. Arch Sex Behav 1997;26(4):343–58.
24. Kruesi MJ, Fine S, Valladares L, et al. Paraphilias: a double-blind crossover comparison of clomipramine versus desipramine. Arch Sex Behav 1992;21(6): 587–93.

25. Lee R, Coccaro E. The neuropharmacology of criminality and aggression. Can J Psychiatry 2001;46(1):35–44.
26. Leo RJ, Kim KY. Clompiramine treatment of paraphilias in elderly demented patients. J Geriatr Psychiatry Neurol 1995;8(2):123–4.
27. Selah FM, Berlin FS. Sex hormones, neurotransmitters, and psychopharmacological treatments in men with paraphilic disorders. J Child Sex Abus 2003;12(3/4):233–53.
28. Bradford JM. The neurobiology, neuropharmacology, and pharmacological treatment of the paraphilas and compulsive sexual behavior. Can J Psychiatry 2001; 46(1):26–34.
29. Bradford JM. The role of serotonin in the future of forensic psychiatry. Bull Am Acad Psychiatry Law 1996;24(1):57–72.
30. Von Krafft-Ebing R. Psychopathia sexualis. New York: Bantam Books; 1969.
31. Blair CD, Lanyon RI. Exhibitionism: etiology and treatment. Psychol Bull 1981; 89(4):439–63.
32. Rahman Q. The neurodevelopment of human sexual orientation. Neurosci Biobehav Rev 2005;29(7):1057–66.
33. Fagan PJ, Wise TN, Schmidt CW, et al. Pedophilia. JAMA 2002;228(19):2458–65.
34. Berlin FS. Pedophilia: when is a difference a disorder? Arch Sex Behav 2002; 31(6):479–80.
35. Berlin FS. Child psychiatrist. In: Spitzer RL, Gibbon M, Spodol AE, et al, editors. DSM-III-R case book: a learning companion to the diagnostic and statistical manual of mental disorders. 3rd edition.. Washington, DC: American Psychiatric Press; 1989. p. 135–7 [revised].
36. Cullington CJ. Psychosurgery: national commission issues surprisingly favorable report. Science 1976;194:299–301.
37. Roeder FD, Muller D, Orthner H. The sterotaxic treatment of pedophilic homosexuality and other sexual deviations. In: Hitchcock E, Laitinen L, Vaernet K, editors. Psychosurgery. Springfield (IL): Thomas; 1972. p. 87–111.
38. Gaffney GR, Berlin FS. Is there a hypothalamic-pituitary-gonadal dysfunction in pedophilia? Br J Psychiatry 1984;145:657–60.
39. Maes M, DeVos N, Van Hunsel F. Pedophilia is accompanied by increased plasma concentrations of catecholamines, in particular epinephrine. Psychiatry Res 2001;103:43–9.
40. Kirenskaya-Berus AV, Tkachenko AA. Characteristic features of EEG spectral characteristics in persons with deviant sexual behavior. Hum Physiol 2003; 29(3):278–87.
41. Blanchard R, Kuban ME, Klassen P, et al. Self-reported head injuries before and after age 13 in pedophilic and nonpedophilic men referred for clinical assessment. Arch Sex Behav 2003;32(6):573–81.
42. Burns JM, Swerdlow RH. Right orbitofrontal tumor with pedophilia symptom and constructional apraxia sign. Arch Neurol 2003;60(3):437–40.
43. Schiffer B, Peschel T, Paul T, et al. Structural brain abnormalities in the frontostriatal system and cerebellum in pedophilia. J Psychiatr Res 2007;41(9):753–62.
44. Phillips-Farfán BV, Lemus AE, Fernández-Guasti A. Increased estrogen receptor alpha inmunoreactivity in the forebrain of sexually satiated rats. Horm Behav 2007;51(3):328–34.
45. Spinella M. The role of prefrontal systems in sexual behavior. Int J Neurosci 2007; 117(3):369–85.
46. Hernández-González M, Prieto-Beracoechea CA, Arteaga-Silva M, et al. Different functionality of the medial and orbital prefrontal cortex during a sexually motivated task in rats. Physiol Behav 2007;90(2/3):450–8.

47. Auger AP. Steroid receptor control of reproductive behavior. Horm Behav 2004; 45(3):168–72.
48. Nedergaard P. Cholinergic, noradrenergic, and GABAergic control of sexual behavior. Scandinavian Journal of Sexology 2000;3(1):3–11.
49. Pfaus JG, Kippen TE, Coria-Avila G. What can animal models tell us about human sexual response? Annu Rev Sex Res 2003;14:1–63.
50. Hiller J. Speculations in the links between feelings, emotions, and sexual behavior: are vasopressin and oxytocin involved? Sexual and Relationship Therapy 2004;19(4):393–429.
51. Curtis JT, Liu Y, Aragona BJ, et al. Dopamine and monogamy. Brain Res 2006; 1126(1):76–90.
52. McGaugh JL, Weinberger NM, Whalen RE. Psychobiology: the biological bases of behavior. San Francisco (CA): Freeman; 1966.
53. Tinbergen N. The curious behavior of the stickleback. In: McGaugh JL, Weinberger NM, Whalen RE, editors. Psychobiology: the biological bases of behavior. San Francisco (CA): Freeman; 1966. p. 5–9.
54. Foss BM. New horizons in psychology. Baltimore (MD): Penguin Books; 1966. 185–208.
55. Goy R, McEwen BS. Sexual differentiation of the brain. Cambridge (MA): MIT Press; 1977.
56. Miller JA. A song for the female finch. Sci News 1980;117:58–9.
57. Money J. Clinical aspects of prenatal steroidal action on sexually dimorphic behavior. In: Sawyer CH, Gorski RA, editors. Steroid hormones and brain function. Berkeley (CA): University of California Press; 1971. p. 325–38.
58. Fisher AE. Behavior as a function of certain neurobiochemical events: current trends in psychobiological theory. Pittsburgh (PA): University of Pittsburgh Press; 1960. p. 70–86.
59. Lorenz KZ. King Solomon's ring: new light on animal ways. New York: Thomas & Chromwell; 1952.
60. Baker P, Telfer MA, Richardson CE, et al. Chromosome errors in men with antisocial behaviors. JAMA 1970;214(5):869–78.
61. Mac Lusky NJ, Naftolin F. Sexual differentiations of the central nervous system. Science 1981;211:1294–303.
62. Meston CM. The neurobiology of sexual function. Arch Gen Psychiatry 2000; 57(11):1012–30.
63. Eher R. Social information processed self-perceived aggression in relation to brain abnormalities in a sample of incarcerated sexual offenders. J Psychol Human Sex 2000;11(3):37–47.
64. Physicians' desk reference. Engel K, editor. Montvale (NJ): Thompson PDR; 2007. p. 2573–76.
65. Levine S. Sex differences in the brain. In: McGaugh JL, Weinberger NM, Whalen RE, editors. Psychobiology: the biological basis of behavior. San Francisco (CA): Freeman; 1966. p. 76–81.
66. Adkins EK. Hormonal basis of sexual differentiation in Japanese quail. J Comp Physiol Psychol 1973;89(1):61–71.
67. McEwen BS. Prenatal determination of adult sexual behavior. Lancet 1981; 11(81):1149–50.
68. Nielsen J. Gender role identity and sexual behavior in persons with sex chromosome aberrations. Dan Med Bull 1972;17(8):269–75.
69. Wilson JD, George FW, Griffin JE. The hormonal control of sexual development. Science 1981;211:1278–84.

70. Ehrhardt AA, Epstein R, Money J. Fetal androgens and female gender identity in the early treated adreno-genital syndrome. Johns Hopkins Med J 1980;122:160–7.

71. Ehrhardt AA, Baker SW. Prenatal androgen exposure and adolescent behavior. In: Porter R, Wheelan J, editors. Sex hormones and behavior. Amsterdam: Excerpta Medica; 1979. p. 41–50.

72. Ehrhardt AA, Money J. Progesterone Induced hermaphrodism: IQ and psychosexual identity in a study of ten girls. J Sex Res 1967;3:83–100.

73. Ehrhardt AA, Grisanti GC, Meyer-Bahlburg HF. Prenatal exposure to medroxyprogesterone acetate (MPA) in girls. Psychoneuroendocrinology 1977;2:391–8.

74. Yalom JP, Green R, Fisk N. Prenatal exposure to female hormones: effect on psychosexual development in boys. Arch Gen Psychiatry 1973;28:554–61.

75. Meyer-Bahlburg HF, Grisanti GC, Ehrhardt AA. Prenatal effects of sex hormones on human male behavior: medroxyprogesterone acetate (MPA). Psychoneuroendocrinology 1977;2:383–90.

76. Spinella M. Hypersexuality and dysecutive syndrome after a thalamic infarct. Int J Neurosci 2004;114(12):1581–90.

77. Physicians' desk reference. Engel K, editor. Montvale (NJ): Thompson PDR; 2007. p. 859–62.

78. Rao V, Handel S, Vaishnavi S, et al. Psychiatric sequelae of traumatic brain injury: a case report. Am J Psychiatry 2007;164(5):728–35.

79. Frost JJ, Wagner HN, Dannals RF, et al. Imaging of opiate receptors in human brain by positron tomography. J Comput Assist Tomogr 1985;9:231–6.

80. Phelps M. Positron computed studies of cerebral glucose metabolism in man: theory and application in nuclear medicine. Semin Nucl Med 1981;11:32–49.

81. Ter-Pogosoian MM, Raichle MM, Sobel BE. Positron emission tomography. Sci Am 1980;10:169–81.

82. Redouté J, Stoléru S, Grégoíre M, et al. Brain processing of visual sexual stimuli in human males. Hum Brain Mapp 2000;11(3):162–77.

83. Stark R, Schienle A, Girod C, et al. Erotic and disgust-inducing pictures: differences in the hemodynamic responses of the brain. Biol Psychiatry 2005;70(1):19–29.

84. Amin Z, Canili T, Epperson C. Effect of estrogen–serotonin interactions on mood and cognition. Behav Cogn Neurosci Rev 2005;4(1):43–58.

85. Karoma S, Lecours AR, Leroux J, et al. Areas of brain activation in males and females during viewing of erotic film excerpts. Hum Brain Mapp 2002;16(1):1–13.

86. Hamann S, Herman RA, Nolan CL, et al. Men and women differ in amygdala response to visual sexual stimuli. Nat Neurosci 2004;7(4):411–6.

87. Hostege G, Georgiadis JR, Paans AM, et al. Brain activation during human male ejaculation. J Neurosci 2003;23(27):9185–93.

88. Pert CB. Type I and Type II opiate receptor distribution in brain: what does it tell us? In: Martin JB, Reichlin S, Biche KL, editors. Neurosecretion and brain peptides. New York: Raven; 1981. p. 117–31.

89. Cushman P. Sexual behavior in heroin addiction and methadone maintenance: correlation with plasma luteinizing hormone. N Y State J Med 1972;72:1261–5.

90. Sirinathsinghji DJ, Whittington PE, Andsley A, et al. Beta-endorphin regulates lordosis in female rats by modulating Lh-Rh release. Nature 1983;301(6):62–4.

91. McIntosh TK, Vallano ML, Barfield RJ. Effects of morphine, beta-endorphin, and naloxone on catacholamine levels and sexual behavior in the male rat. Pharmacol Biochem Behav 1980;13:435–41.

92. Gessa GL, Paglietti E, Quarantolli BP. Induction of copulatory behavior in sexually inactive rats by naloxone. Science 1979;204(13):203–4.

93. Miren SM, Meyer RE, Mendelson JH, et al. Opiate use and sexual function. Am J Psychiatry 1980;137:909–15.
94. Szechtman H, Hershkowitz M, Simantov R. Sexual behavior decreases pain sensitivity and stimulates endogenous opiates in male rats. Eur J Pharmacol 1981;70:279–85.
95. Frost JJ, Mayberg HS, Berlin FS, et al. Alteration in brain opiate receptor binding in man following arousal using C-11 carfentinil and positron emission tomography. Proceedings of the 33rd Annual Meeting of the Society of Nuclear Medicine. J Nucl Med 1986;27(6):1027.

Sexual Arousal Patterns: Normal and Deviant

Gene G. Abel, MD[a,b,c,d,]*, Latricia Coffey, MD[c,e],
Candice A. Osborn, MA, LPC[a]

KEYWORDS

• Paraphilias • Etiology • Fetish • Childhood • Viewing time

The origin and development of sexual arousal in humans has been discussed in the literature for years, long before the well-known publications of Sigmund Freud. A variety of views existed within the scientific community regarding what is considered normal sexual development and how it occurs.[1,2] At the same time, a great deal of discussion has focused on defining what is considered sexually deviant and how we, as a society, should deal with it. There has recently been debate about whether or not the paraphilias (deviant sexual interests and behaviors) constitute psychopathology at all.[3–5] Just as there is discussion about whether sexually deviant interests and behaviors should constitute mental illness, there is also debate about whether they should even be considered "abnormal."

Some sexual behaviors that were once deemed deviant by society and the medical field have been recently accepted into the mainstream with advancements in our understanding and our theories about how sexuality occurs. For example, both homosexuality and masturbation were historically proscribed or considered aberrant in Western society. Conceptualizations of both have dramatically changed over the years. Given the changes in attitude, both scientific and social, there are those who argue that other practices currently deemed deviant will, similarly, eventually be

Dr. Abel is president of Abel Screening, Inc., an organization that develops and manufactures products that incorporate Viewing Time Measurement and questionnaires for the assessment of potential sexual offenders.

[a] Behavioral Medicine Institute of Atlanta, 1401 Peachtree Street, Suite 140, Atlanta, GA 30309, USA

[b] Emory University School of Medicine, 1365 Clifton Road NE, Atlanta, GA 30322, USA

[c] Morehouse School of Medicine, 720 Westview Drive SW, Atlanta, GA 30310, USA

[d] Abel Screening, Inc., 1401 Peachtree Street, Suite 120, Atlanta, GA 30309, USA

[e] Laurel Heights Hospital, 934 Briarcliff Road NE, Atlanta, GA 30306, USA

* Corresponding author. Behavioral Medicine Institute of Atlanta, 1401 Peachtree Street, Suite 140, Atlanta, GA 30309.

E-mail address: geneabel@earthlink.com (G.G. Abel).

Psychiatr Clin N Am 31 (2008) 643–655
doi:10.1016/j.psc.2008.07.001
0193-953X/08/$ – see front matter © 2008 published by Elsevier Inc.

psych.theclinics.com

embraced as "normal" and generally acceptable. Such is the logic that groups such as the North American Man/Boy Love Association[6] and the now defunct Rene Guyon Society use to endorse sexual relationships between adults and children.

Currently, the scientific community classifies deviant sexual interest under the category of paraphilias: recurrent, intense, sexually arousing fantasies, urges, or behaviors generally involving (1) nonhuman objects, (2) the suffering or humiliation of oneself or one's partner, or (3) children or other nonconsenting persons. Changes in the *Diagnostic and Statistical Manual of Mental Disorders* versions over the years reflect concern about the line between an individual's sexual interests and his or her behavior. The *Diagnostic and Statistical Manual of Mental Disorders, Revised Third Edition* defined paraphilias, under criterion A, as recurrent, intense sexual urges and arousing fantasies (with no reference to behaviors), involving 1, 2, and 3 above. Criterion B stated the diagnosis was made only when the urges caused the person marked distress or if he acted on them. Additionally, the severity specifiers all related to how often the person acted on the urges. However, *Diagnostic and Statistical Manual of Mental Disorders, Fourth Edition* added the word "behaviors" to criterion A and eliminated the latter part of criterion B, thus allowing diagnosis only if the person suffered clinically significant distress, regardless of whether he had acted on the urges. Now, with *Diagnostic and Statistical Manual of Mental Disorders, Fourth Edition, Text Revision*, the diagnosis for certain paraphilias can once again be made if the person acts on the urges, regardless of the presence of clinical distress. For example, the diagnosis of sexual sadism is made if the person has acted on the urges *or* if they cause marked distress. However, fetishism can only be diagnosed if the urges or behaviors cause significant distress.[7–9]

Although theories abound on deviant arousal patterns in general, much of the recent research has focused specifically on pedophilic interests. Abel and colleagues[10] discuss three of the most popular theories: Psychoanalytic theory states that deviant sexuality is caused by "persistence beyond childhood of earlier forms of sexuality as preferred expressions." Feelings of security with this behavior are preferable to venturing into the unknown (adults), and the ego accepts the unrepressed infantile fantasies. In the cognitive model, distortions are prominent. In studies of sex offenders, the combination of similar character traits with the presence of cognitive distortions allows the offender to continually sexually abuse with minimal regard for the victim. The conditioning and social learning model describes how pairing deviant thoughts and behaviors with a positive reinforcer, orgasm, becomes an *intermittent, variable-ratio enforcement*, the most difficult type to extinguish.[11,12]

Despite advances in technology, expansion of understanding, and changes in morality, certain sexual acts, because of their inherent victimization and harm, will likely remain offensive to Western society. Society in general (except for certain religious and conservative groups) is relatively unconcerned with how an individual chooses to achieve erotic stimulation unless that stimulation acquires a tangible quality and begins to infringe on the rights of others. Therefore, studies about the origin and pattern of deviant sexual arousal and how that arousal moves from fantasy to behavior are important undertakings.

Researchers have discovered that deviant sexual fantasies often lead to deviant sexual behavior.[10,11,13] For example, it is common for convicted sex offenders to describe deviant sexual fantasies that preceded their criminal behavior.[14] Mainly due to fear of potential sexual aggression, society is concerned about what to do with those who are sexually deviant. These fears are in some ways well founded because paraphiliacs make up a significant category of offenders who commit high numbers of sex crimes, usually beginning in adolescence.[10,15]

Determining the exact manner in which an individual's sexual arousal pattern develops is exceedingly difficult because of the complexities of interviewing young children about sexual interest, beginning with the child's lack of communication skills to describe even the concept of sexual interest. A further problem with clarifying the developmental elements of sexual interest is that the predominant data source has been retrospective memory, which has several limitations, particularly on questions of validity. One method of attempting to clarify when, how, and where sexual interest develops is to examine a sexual interest that is so unique or unusual that it stands out in the individual's memory. Through this tracking, it is possible to see how the individual attempts to blend his unusual arousal patterns into a "normal" sex life. For example, the literature includes studies in which transvestic fetishists (cross-dressers) recall being dressed in girls' clothing by female family members who expressed delight or amusement and then later masturbating and incorporating the fetish objects (girls' clothing) into their sexual fantasies.[16]

EARLY AROUSAL PATTERNS

"Sexual" behavior occurs in infants as they touch and stimulate their genitals. However, not much is known about the extent to which a child seeks out others or external stimuli for erotic gratification because there is little in the scientific literature about sexual arousal patterns in school-age children. The subject is problematic to broach, in part because young children often do not have the language skills to accurately communicate their sexual interests and behavior, but also because of parental and societal resistance to discussing sexual issues with children. It has been observed that children engage in masturbatory and exploratory activities with themselves and peers, but there is little to suggest that sexual fantasy occurs in this age group. As a child develops into an adolescent, sexual thoughts probably acquire erotic meaning through classical conditioning. Through stimulus pairing, the event/stimulus is associated with arousal, culminating in orgasm and thus acquires erotic potential. If the individual cognitively decides the sexual stimulus is good and favorable, its arousal value is enhanced; if he or she feels the arousal was negative, it may be inhibited.

It is also necessary to accurately perceive physiologic arousal and attach it to the correct emotion. If physiologic arousal is inaccurately perceived as intense attraction or sexual behavior, rather than as anxiety, guilt, or other confusing emotions that may contribute to stimulation, it can begin to elicit sexual arousal. The individual may then continue to seek out similar stimuli for sexual arousal. Attention is another necessary component of sexual stimulation. An indicator of emotional attachment to a sexual stimulus is the level of attention directed at the object. Those with deviant sexual interest patterns show increased attention to their desired objects, similar to those with normal sexual interest. These attentional mechanisms involve implicit and explicit sexual memory, as well as regulatory roles. First, physiological arousal occurs as described above, then attentional mechanisms are activated to allow conscious appraisal of the arousal as sexual: "This thing is causing sexual arousal." Attention to internal and external sexual cues is required, or the sexual response will stop.[14]

Deviant interests frequently develop very early and sometimes continue into adulthood. Others are extinguished or sublimated into behaviors acceptable to partners. Yet other interests remain secret, a factor that in itself is somewhat sexually stimulating and contributes to the escalation of the arousal. There is little prospective data about adolescents with paraphilic interest. Most of the data is retrospective after the individual has progressed to criminally acting upon his deviant sexual interests.[15]

The six cases described here, chosen from a large body of similar cases, reflect how the individual's life experiences form the basis for the development of unusual arousal patterns. In each case, the individual's fascination with the arousing fetish object has been present for as long as he can remember, allowing the authors to track this unique arousal pattern through early life and examine the attempts to blend fetish interest into adult sexual interactions. We cannot be certain that the development of these unique sexual interests is similar to how "normal" sexual interests develop. However, because these unique sexual interests can be clearly followed, these cases provide an excellent opportunity to track each individual's efforts at integrating them into adult sexual life and, in some cases, into sexual interactions with a partner. These cases provide further evidence that deviant arousal patterns can develop early in childhood, predating identified sexuality, often by years. Conditioning and stimulus-pairing reinforce the arousal through the pleasures of masturbation and orgasm and often culminate in the individual acting on the arousing images/fantasies. Trauma and other events can impact the development of sexual interests. Normal sexual arousal patterns likely develop in a similar pattern.

CASE STUDIES

To objectively measure the patients' sexual interest pattern, all of the patients described in the following cases underwent the Visual Reaction Time (VRT) measure, part of the Abel Assessment for Sexual Interest.[16–18] In general, the stimuli included 160 images that depict a frontal view of the individual in a bathing suit or lingerie without depictions of sexual activity or sexual arousal. The images portray males and females of Caucasian and African American ethnicity in two age groups: adults over age 21, and prepubescent school-age children. The specific categories are as follows: adult females, adult females–black, adult males, adult males–black, young females, young females–black, young males, and young males–black. Additional images portray six types of non–child-related paraphilic sexual behavior: exhibitionism targeting adult females, sadomasochism targeting adult females, sadomasochism targeting adult males, frotteurism targeting adult females, voyeurism targeting adult females, fetishism (lingerie), and neutral slides of landscapes. For some of the cases described below, the images in the frotteurism category were replaced with images of objects consistent with the individual's reported, specific fetish interests. The amount of time the patient views each slide (measured in milliseconds) reflects the degree of sexual interest he has in that particular category. The stimulus set includes seven images (photographic slides) in each category, and the individual's average viewing time in each category is compared with his average viewing time in the other categories (Z scores).[17]

Mr. Cartoons

Mr. Cartoons, age 18, was referred for an evaluation after he revealed to his pediatrician that he had sexual interest in young girls. He had never been accused of child molestation, and was not under investigation for such behavior. He had normal intelligence, but a very limited social life.

At age 11, he began looking at adult erotica on the Internet and quickly progressed to viewing *hentai*, sexually explicit or pornographic comics and animation produced in Japan, often involving children who are being sexually abused. He began collecting these cartoons, spending up to 12 hours per month looking at and downloading them. He clearly reported that this led to his developing sexual interest in young girls. By age 12, he recognized that thoughts of touching children were highly arousing to him, with a preference for girls 10 to 13 years old. He also reported that he had developed sexual interest in his 8-year-old female neighbor. He was able to successfully conceal his sexual interests because he has had no partners and the object of his interest primarily existed in fantasy (ie, the Internet).

He reported that 50% of his masturbatory fantasies were of young girls, a small percentage were of him being a young girl having sex with a male, and the rest involving adult females. He indicated that the more he looked at the cartoons, the greater his interest in touching young girls in the real world became. He denied being abused or ever abusing children. By showing images of various males and females to Mr. Cartoon, his sexual interest in young girls and adult females was substantiated.

He was reluctant to tell others about his sexual interest in young girls, fearing that he would be arrested or labeled as "sick" or perverted. His peers knew that he looked at *hentai* cartoons and their response was that he was "gross." When a relative became the victim of child sexual abuse, his family questioned Mr. Cartoons as to whether he had ever been abused. At that time, he told a family member that he had looked at some "sex cartoons" in the past, but falsely said that he no longer did, although he continued to look at *hentai*.

In *hentai*, many of the characters are of ambiguous gender and the sex acts can include children with children, children with adults, or children with creatures, including acts that are physically impossible. Of note, Mr. Cartoons acknowledged not feeling that he was masculine and that he hated being a male. It is possible that this gender confusion fueled his interest in these cartoons, or vice versa.

Fortunately, Mr. Cartoons willingly sought help, despite his fear of being called "sick." He was under no pressure to reveal his view of the etiology of his sexual interest in children and was very clear that, before looking at the *hentai* cartoons, he had no sexual interest in children. The Internet provided him access to adult erotica but he quickly moved to Japanese child pornography cartoons that required no age confirmation to view or download.

This case demonstrates how a common Internet activity, such as viewing animated cartoons, can easily lead to exposure to adult material in the same child-friendly medium and emphasizes the importance of parents knowing what their children are viewing on the Internet. It also highlights holes in the system for preventing children from gaining access to child pornography, in the form of these cartoons. Unlike the other cases below, Mr. Cartoons has never been involved in a physical relationship with another person. Similar to the following cases, he felt that his behavior was perverted and that more people would seek help if they were not afraid of being vilified. His social discomfort and lack of experience in dating peers, coupled with his sexual interest in children, led him to a dead end in terms of expressing his sexual interest. Continued masturbation to sexual fantasies with children had already increased his risk of molesting children, while his fear, anxiety, and lack of social skills blocked him from developing a prosocial sexual life.

Mr. Feet

Mr. Feet, a mental health worker in his 40s, was referred after being arrested and charged with aggravated sexual battery of a girl under age 5, after he picked up a young girl, rolled her around on his lap, and played with her feet. When he stood up, a spot of pre-ejaculate was observed on his pants. He was reported, investigated, and eventually arrested.

He stated that when he was 3 years old and lying on a changing table, the female caring for him was playing with and smelling his feet as if it were a pleasurable and fun activity for her. The following year, a girl slightly older than him stuck her bare toe into his mouth; he was puzzled as to why she was doing this, felt dominated, and did not enjoy the experience. From that point on, he reported having a sustained interest in children's feet and, by age 10, was fantasizing about smelling young children's feet, both boys and girls. As a child, he would look at other children's feet and, when he began dating in high school, he was particularly attracted to the feet of the females he dated.

His preoccupation with feet continued throughout his limited dating history. Being exceedingly passive, he did not specifically play with or smell the feet of his dates, but became quite aroused if they rubbed their bare feet against his back, under the guise of receiving a type of foot back-rub. He was most attracted to smelling feet, scratching feet, and having partners remove their shoes and socks and push their feet against his body. He reported that directly touching feet was actually less erotic than these activities. He denied being sexually attracted to young children and denied ever fondling a child's genital's for sexual gratification, but did report that smelling children's feet was highly erotic. When asked why he selected children's feet to smell, feel, and play with, he said that society is accustomed to seeing adults touch and play with the feet of children and actually views it as a fun experience for the children. However, similar behavior with an adult partner could be seen as perverted.

He reported that 20% of his masturbatory fantasies were of sexual experiences with adult females, while the other 80% were of smelling or playing with children's feet. He admitted that during the incident for which he was arrested, removing the young girl's shoes and socks was highly erotic. This was consistent with his report that he found smelling the feet of 3- to 8-year-old boys or girls particularly arousing.

Two steps were taken to substantiate the validity of his self-report, since there was concern that he might be sexually attracted to children and was using his partialism (a fetish for parts of the body) as a diversion to avoid the diagnosis of pedophilia. A polygraph examination confirmed that, as an adult, he never asked children to take off their clothes or to touch his genitals for sexual pleasure, and that he never touched children's genitals. He also underwent VRT measurement, in which he was additionally shown seven images of adult women's feet. Although he minimized his self-reported arousal to the women's feet, indicating they were actually sexually repulsive to him, VRT showed his sexual interest in these images to be equivalent to his objectively recorded sexual interest in adolescent and adult females. He showed no evidence of sexual interest in images of preschool or grade-school females or males from a total of 56 slides depicting underage children.

Mr. Feet was well educated and throughout his career had worked with facilities for child care, families, and the disabled. Because of his intellectual acuity, he was able to successfully conceal, yet act upon, his sexual interests for years. This case demonstrates how benign activities at an early age, such as sensing an adult's enjoyment while touching his feet paired with negative emotions (feeling dominated), can have a profound impact on an individual's subsequent sexual interests. This individual's sexual fascination with feet clearly preceded his defining the experience as sexual and emerged far anterior to masturbatory activities. As he developed, his attachment to children's feet generalized to his attachment to the feet of adult females and he attempted to incorporate this sexual interest into playing with the feet of his adult partners. However, he found it impossible to approach his adult sexual partners in a forthright manner about his partialism. He subsequently gravitated to opportunities where smelling and touching the feet of others could go unnoticed (ie, by touching the feet of children). Were it not for the pre-ejaculate seen on his pants, his activity would have gone unnoticed.

Mr. Feet had reached a precarious position in terms of his sexual life. He was unsuccessful at convincing sexual partners to incorporate touching and smelling of feet into their sexual interaction. At the same time, his ability to incorporate his partialism into apparent benign tickling of children's feet was increasing his risk to extend his sexual interest in children beyond their feet and become involved in child sexual abuse.

Mr. Balloons

Mr. Balloons, an 18-year-old mildly retarded male, was arrested after repeatedly walking into department stores, asking sales clerks to blow up balloons, and masturbating while watching them blow up the balloons from 30 or 40 ft away. He was accompanied to the assessment by his father, who gave a clear history of his son's experience with balloons. While attending a church party at age 6, where balloons were decorations, some of the balloons popped. Mr. Balloons became terrified of the sound, ran from the church, and had to be tackled before he could be stopped. Starting at that time, he avoided situations where there were loud noises or balloons.

When he was a young teenager, his parents were surprised to find balloons in his room since previously he had conspicuously avoided them. He recounted that, around this time, he began to masturbate while blowing up balloons. He next brought younger friends over to have them blow up balloons while he masturbated near them. Because he was in special classes in school and was socially inept, he never dated. However, he began taking balloons into stadiums at sports events and asking women to blow them up while he masturbated from a distance. This extended to a variety of settings in which his requests were seen as peculiar, obnoxious behavior by a mildly retarded individual. However, his requests became more public, as did his masturbation while watching women blow up the balloons. Ultimately, this behavior led to his numerous arrests and referral.

To objectively evaluate Mr. Balloons' sexual interests, pictures were taken of women blowing up balloons of various sizes, as well as pictures of a number of deflated balloons. These images were incorporated into visual reaction time measurement and, as expected, VRT showed his sexual interest in balloons to be far in excess of his interest in adult or adolescent females (**Fig. 1**).

This case demonstrates another etiologic process for the development of sexual interest, namely, a traumatic event. Popping of balloons produced fear, followed by avoidance of the feared object or sound, followed by use of the feared object to become sexually aroused (which was likely the result of incorrectly attributing the arousal associated with fear/anxiety as erotic arousal). The subjective experience of fearfulness consequently diminished and was replaced by sexual arousal associated with the feared object, reinforced through masturbation and orgasm (so-called "identification with the aggressor"). Mr. Balloons' lack of social skills and dating experiences, combined with his lower intellect, blocked his efforts to have the mainstream sexual experiences of high school students. However, his growing sexual interest in balloons, years of masturbating while blowing up balloons, and interest in watching others blow up balloons became impassable obstacles to sexual activity with a partner. His displays of masturbating while watching adult women blow up balloons allowed society no other choice than to arrest him. He appears stuck in an impossible situation: strong persistent sexual interest in an activity that cannot be subsumed into sexual activity with others.

Mr. Rings

Mr. Rings, a man in his 30s, sought out evaluation for his preoccupation with women's rings and excessive spending on lap dances at strip bars. He had no legal charges and was not under investigation for inappropriate behavior.

He reported remembering sitting on his aunt's lap at age 4 and looking at her rings that had wide bands and diamonds. Since that time, he has become more and more

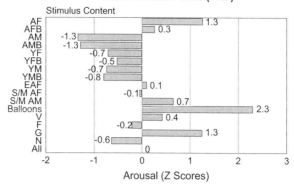

Fig. 1. VRT results for Mr. Balloons presented in the form of Z scores. The patient's Z score to images of women blowing up balloons (2.3) was significantly higher than his Z scores to all other categories of sexual images. AF, adult females; AFB, adult females–black; AM, adult males; AMB, adult males–black; EAF, exhibitionism targeting adult females; F, fetishism (lingerie); G, gross (unattractive pictures of skin lesions); N, neutral slides of landscapes; S/M AF, sadomasochism targeting adult females; S/M AM, sadomasochism targeting adult males; V, voyeurism targeting adult females; YF, young females; YFB, young females–black; YM, young males; YMB, young males–black.

preoccupied with women's rings, especially wedding bands 10 to 12 mm wide. By ages 10 to 13, he was masturbating three times per day to fantasies of women's rings, and by age 17 he began looking at pornography. He reported being attracted mostly to married women, perhaps because they were wearing the rings that interested him the most. He married in his early 20s and found it highly arousing to twirl his wife's wedding rings around her finger during intercourse. He insisted on buying all of her rings himself.

He later bought three video cameras and would spend 6 hours a weekend videotaping various women's rings. He was interested in the rings on the women's hands, not their faces or bodies. He was successful under the guise that his wife had lost her wedding ring and he wanted to videotape rings he felt would be a good replacement. However, many of the women did not know they were being videotaped.

One year before his evaluation, he began going to strip bars and became emotionally involved with a stripper. He asked her to wear rings during her performances for him. He typically spent $100 to $300 per month at the strip bar, but one weekend spent over $2000, which precipitated new marital conflict, refueled former disputes, and led to his referral for assessment. He brought 6 hours of edited video tapes of women's hands adorned with rings to his assessment. He reported that his routine was to edit the videos at home to include only the rings that were most erotic to him, and then masturbate to these images.

At that time, 95% of his sexual fantasies were about women's rings and less than 5% of his fantasies were about adult females, primarily strippers. VRT measurement comparing images of rings versus images of adult and adolescent females, heterosexual and lesbian couples, and other categories of paraphilias, clearly showed his greatest sexual interest was to the images of rings, which was consistent with his self-report (**Fig. 2**).

Mr. Rings' sexual interest in rings was initiated by an early-age sensation of excitement and pleasure to a repeated experience involving wedding bands and diamond

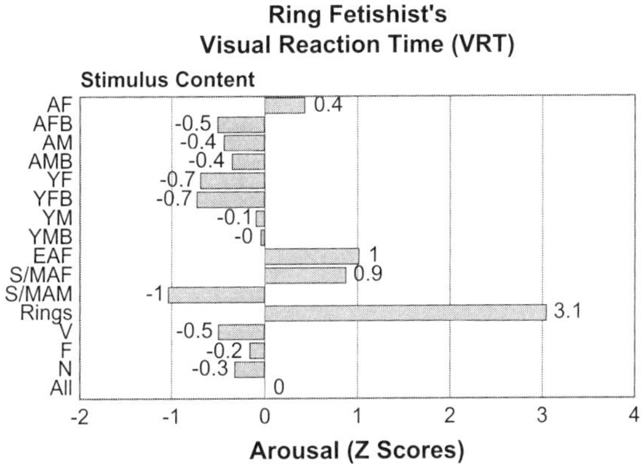

Fig. 2. VRT results for Mr. Rings are presented in the form of Z scores. This patient's Z score to images of women's rings (3.1) was significantly higher than his Z scores to all other categories of sexual mages. AF, adult females; AFB, adult females–black; AM, adult males; AMB, adult males–black; EAF, exhibitionism targeting adult females; F, fetishism (lingerie); N, neutral slides of landscapes; S/M AF, sadomasochism targeting adult females; S/M AM, sadomasochism targeting adult males; V, voyeurism targeting adult females; YF, young females; YFB, young females–black; YM, young males; YMB, young males–black.

rings. This fascination with rings occurred far anterior to his developing a sexual drive. When he began to masturbate, he fantasized about images of rings that he had seen and, with the advent of video camcorders, he was able to collect masturbatory material under the guise of trying to select a replacement for his wife's lost wedding ring. Again, we see object fascination before the development of sexual interest and then a masturbatory pattern reinforcing the fetish hundreds of times. Mr. Rings' fetish then was incorporated into sexual activity with his wife, as he twirled her wedding ring around her finger during intercourse. Because he was of average intelligence and reasonably well socialized, he was able to use technology to successfully conceal his sexual interest from others while amassing video footage of rings that were extremely arousing to him. Interestingly, he made no attempts to establish a sexual relationship with any of the women whose rings he recorded on video. It was only after his drive to spend money on a stripper depleted his finances that the extent of his sexual interest came to the attention of a psychiatrist.

Mr. Rings attempted to incorporate his fetish interest into his sexual activity with his partner, but he was only partially successful in that his wife realized that his interest in an inanimate object, her rings, was stronger than his sexual interest in her. As their marriage progressed, bigger arguments ensued, not only about his preoccupation with rings, but also his treating her more as a sexual object than an intimate partner. As his sexual behavior extended outside of his marriage, his preoccupation with rings went with it and was tolerated by the lap dancers that he hired.

Mr. Cigarettes

Mr. Cigarettes, also in his 30s, was referred by his defense attorney after tens of thousands of pictures of women smoking cigarettes were found on his company computer. He had been arrested for misuse of company property.

At age 8, he became interested in smoking by watching his parents and grandparents smoke and he looked forward to being able to smoke when he got older. At age 12, he read a sex education book and began to masturbate. He masturbated to cigarette ads in magazines and found this exceedingly arousing. By age 18, he was masturbating daily, predominantly to images of women smoking, with 90% of his masturbatory fantasies involving images of women smoking.

He married in his 20s, but did not tell his wife of his extensive sexual interest in women smoking because he viewed it as bizarre and thought he would be rejected by his wife for having these desires. By his early 30s, the frequency of sexual intercourse with his wife had declined and he started searching for smoking-related sites on the Internet. He began downloading pictures, stories, or videos of women smoking, especially if the image showed a woman inhaling or exhaling the smoke. These images were subsequently discovered by his wife, who became enraged because of his interest in smoking and his concealment of this aspect of his sexual life. To avoid further detection by his wife, he downloaded these images on his computer at work.

At one point, he tried smoking while masturbating, but he found looking at women smoking to be far more erotic. He was unable to get a full erection while he smoked unless he fantasized about a woman smoking, sharing a cigarette with her, touching her, or her performing fellatio on him while she smoked, holding a cigarette in her hand. Ninety-five percent of his masturbatory fantasies involved women smoking, while 5% involved being sexual with his wife.

To objectively measure Mr. Cigarettes' sexual interest in smoking, images of women smoking were retrieved from the Internet and seven of these images were inserted into the standard VRT set. VRT measurements showed him to have high sexual interest in the images of women smokers, and his self-reported sexual arousal to this category far exceeded other categories of appropriate and inappropriate types of sexual interest. He showed no sexual interest in preschool or grade-school children and had normal arousal to adolescent and adult females.

Mr. Cigarettes' interest in smoking began before what he defined as sexual interest. After viewing stereotypical adult erotica, he promptly shifted to using magazine ads depicting women smoking. Fears that he would be labeled as strange or perverted forced him to conceal his sexual preference and prevented him from consulting with a therapist to help him gain control over his unusual sexual interest. Because he was not intellectually impaired or significantly socially impaired, he could successfully maintain the image of being a traditional heterosexual male, while spending hours downloading smoking materials for masturbatory purposes. He was pleased to find so many similar individuals on the Internet supporting smoking sites because this helped him realize that he was "not alone." He reported that, as his wife's sexual drive decreased, he rapidly increased his masturbation to smoking images. He believed his arousal to women inhaling or exhaling smoke was somehow related to their doing something wrong or harmful to themselves (ie, smoking).

Mr. Cigarettes could not incorporate his wife's smoking into sexual activity because she was a nonsmoker. He splintered off this sexual interest as their sexual activity declined in frequency. Downloading thousands of images was a rich source of new, exciting fantasies that incorporated women smoking. Since it was a fetish for women smoking, and not overtly sexual, it was ignored by his employers, but they did not ignore his using a company computer for noncompany business.

Mr. Spanking

Mr. Spanking was an intellectually disabled man in his 30s who suffered a brain injury at birth. He was referred in the midst of divorcing his intellectually disabled wife because of his demands that spanking each other be a part of their sexual interactions.

He reported that he has been preoccupied with spanking since age 5, when he walked in on his brother being spanked on his bare buttocks by his mother. He reported that this stunned and surprised him, and stated that the experience was "like a dream, like a movie." He was shocked because he did not know what was happening and had never before seen his brother being spanked.

He graduated from high school in special education classes, but had marked difficulty dating because of his intellectual disabilities and his lack of social skills. Because of these deficits, his family closely supervised him. By his early 20s, he began searching the neighborhood newspaper for ads about sadomasochism and spanking and reported that he wanted a 15- to 20-year-old woman to spank him. In sheltered workshop situations, he approached other females with his requests for spanking and subsequently was released from his independent living program.

During his assessment, he also reported that from age 8 to 11, he had sexually abused young boys and young girls, and had exposed himself to young females, including teenagers, grade-school girls, young acquaintances, and relatives. By age 27, he began having spanking sessions, both giving and receiving, with prostitutes he hired. A few years later, he began dating a woman he met in one of his special education classes. He subsequently married her. However, in the process of their sexual interactions, he introduced the idea of one of them spanking the other and her family became so alarmed that they were eventually pressured to divorce.

He reported that 60% of his masturbatory fantasies were of spanking and, surprisingly, thoughts of his father spanking him. VRT measurements confirmed his sexual interest in young girls and boys, and his sexual interest in females being dominated was considerably greater than his sexual interest in adult females without such images.

Once again, this case demonstrates how a strong emotional experience, namely one that is startling, surprising, and stunning, has an impact on the individual's sexual development and causes him to focus on fantasies related to the experience. The object of his focus, spanking, was eventually incorporated into his sexual fantasies and masturbatory behavior. This intellectually disabled man, despite being watched closely by family, was able to incorporate his fantasies into his sex life with prostitutes. Once married, however, he was unsuccessful at blending spanking into his sexual activity with his wife. This failure drew attention to his sadomasochistic interest. However, his ongoing pedophilic interest and repeated inappropriate sexual behaviors with children went unnoticed because there were no complainants.

Mr. Spanking could probably have incorporated spanking activity into his marital relationship but, because of his intellectual disability and that of his wife, their sexual activity was watched closely by her parents who immediately took action leading to their divorce. Spanking is sometimes incorporated into a couple's sexual activity but, in this case, concerns by others about the welfare of his partner blocked this possibility.

SUMMARY

The fetish objects in these case histories were unique enough, and the attraction to the objects strong enough, that the individuals could clearly track their interest from early childhood through adulthood. It is much easier to retrieve remote, explicit memories, such as events (eg, a party where balloons popped) or playing with objects, than to recall the process of sexual development with no distinct markers in the individual's history. Because these distinct experiences predated identified sexuality, became a focus of attention for the individual, and then were incorporated into the individual's sexual interests and masturbatory fantasies, it was possible to accurately track the patterns of sexual arousal. We were also able to clearly identify how these men attempted to blend their deviant interests into sexual relationships with partners and the consequences of their efforts.

If we are to understand how sexual interests develop, a number of obstacles need to be overcome. Sexual interest has to be openly discussed. Parents need to appreciate how the early sexual interests of their children can go awry, contaminate their adult relationships, and lead to problematic lives. Researchers need a means of understanding how to communicate with children about their earliest interests, sexual interests, and sexual behaviors in a nonjudgmental manner. Until then, tracking unusual interests that lead to erotic interests is the first step in the overall process of understanding how sexual interest develops and is assimilated, either successfully or unsuccessfully, into an individual's adult sexual life.

REFERENCES

1. Bullough VL. Children and adolescents as sexual beings: a historical overview. Child Adolesc Psychiatr Clin N Am 2004;13(3):447–59.
2. Serbin LA, Sprafkin CH. A developmental approach: sexuality from infancy through adolescence. In: Geer JH, O'Donohue WT, editors. Theories of human sexuality. New York: Plenum Press; 1987. p. 163–95.
3. Green R. Is pedophilia a mental disorder? Arch Sex Behav 2002;31(6):456–71.
4. Radden J, editor. The Philosophy of psychiatry: a companion. Available at: http://fs.uno.edu/asoble/pages/dsmiv.htm. Accessed July 2007.
5. Suppe F. Classifying sexual disorders: the Diagnostic and Statistical Manual of the American Psychiatric Association. J Homosex 1984;9(4):9–28.
6. Available at: http://nambla.org. Accessed July 2007.
7. American Psychiatric Association. Diagnostic and statistical manual of mental disorders. 3rd (revised) edition. Washington, DC: American Psychiatric Association; 1987.
8. American Psychiatric Association. Diagnostic and statistical manual of mental disorders. 4th edition. Washington, DC: American Psychiatric Association; 1994.
9. American Psychiatric Association. Diagnostic and statistical manual of mental disorders. 4th edition. Washington, DC: American Psychiatric Association; 2000. Text Revision.
10. Abel GG, Osborn CA, Twigg DA. Sexual assault through the life span: adult offenders with juvenile histories. In: Barbaree HE, Marshall WL, Laws DR, editors. The juvenile sex offender. New York: Guilford Publications; 1993. p. 104–16.
11. Abel GG, Blanchard EB. The role of fantasy in the treatment of sexual deviation. Arch Gen Psychiatry 1974;30(4):467–75.
12. Laws DR, Marshall WL. A conditioning theory of the etiology and maintenance of deviant sexual preference and behavior. In: Marshall WL, Laws DR, Barbaree HE, editors. Handbook of sexual assault: issues, theories, and treatment of the offender. New York: Plenum; 1990. p. 209–29.
13. Leitenberg H, Henning K. Sexual fantasy. Psychol Bull 1995;117(3):469–96.
14. Scott AA, Reddon JR, Burke AR. Sexual fantasies of adolescent male sex offenders in residential treatment: a descriptive study. Arch Sex Behav 2005; 34(2):231–9.
15. Zolondek SC, Abel GG, Northey WF, et al. The self-reported behaviors of juvenile sexual offenders. J Interpers Violence 2001;16(1):73–85.
16. Schott RL. The childhood and family dynamics of transvestites. Arch Sex Behav 1995;24(3):309–27.

17. Abel GG, Jordan A, Hand CG, et al. Classification models of child molestation utilizing the Abel Assessment for sexual interest™. Child Abuse Negl 2001;25(5): 703–18.
18. Abel GG, Wiegel M. Visual reaction time: development, theory, empirical evidence and beyond. In: Saleh FM, Grudzinskas AJ, Bradford JM, editors. Sex offenders: identification, risk assessment, treatment, and legal issues. New York: Oxford University Press, in press.

Treatment of Sexually Compulsive Adolescents

James Gerber, PhD

KEYWORDS

- Sexual addiction • Sexual compulsivity • Adolescent sexuality
- Treatment of sexual addiction

Various authors have discussed society's contradictory treatment of sexuality.[1,2] On the one hand, although it has been more than 100 years since Freud enlightened Western society about childhood sexuality, children are still kept relatively ignorant about sex. There is rarely any comprehensive teaching of children to help them anticipate and understand their sexual responses. On the other hand, every adolescent is exposed to a barrage of differing messages about sexual behavior from politicians, clergy, television, music, movies, and so forth. Messages from the conservative spectrum of society promote abstinence and traditional religious values. While not all of these present sexuality as evil, or as urges to be suppressed, they do promote rigid guidelines of acceptable behavior.

Adolescents are also exposed to cultural messages that seem to promote hedonism. Implicit and explicit messages about sexuality often objectify women and present an expectation of "hypermasculinity" for males. The two messages portrayed offer polarities. Information about intimacy, responsibility, and realistic sexual encounters is largely absent. Still, individuals are expected to emerge from adolescence with a healthy sexual maturity and a capacity for intimacy.

This is the cultural context in which we consider the term "sexually compulsive adolescent." This term itself might have different meanings to different people. Typically, the term would refer to male adolescents and illegal sexual behaviors. In the past 25 years this population has received considerable attention reflected in the media coverage of sexual crimes, the creation of laws to contain those deemed "sexually dangerous persons," and the development of treatment programs for this population. These trends are based on assumptions that tend to cast the abusive youth as a young adult offender, a predator who is resistant to change.

Letourneau[3] describes the movement toward harsher treatment of adolescent sex offenders to be based on three false assumptions: that there is a epidemic of juveniles committing sex offenses, that juvenile offenders are more like adult sex offenders than

Castlewood Treatment Center, 800 Holland Road, Ballwin, MO 63021, USA
E-mail address: jmgerber@yahoo.com

Psychiatr Clin N Am 31 (2008) 657–669
doi:10.1016/j.psc.2008.06.006
0193-953X/08/$ – see front matter © 2008 published by Elsevier Inc.

psych.theclinics.com

other juvenile delinquents, and that in the absence of specific treatment, juvenile sex offenders are at high risk to re-offend. The author states that the research bears out none of these assumptions. In addition, these assumptions ignore the developmental factors present in adolescence.

Further, sexually abusive males are likely to not be sexually compulsive. For example, in a research study on incarcerated adult offenders, Marshall and Marshall[4] found 35% of the incarcerated population to be sexually compulsive whereas only 12.5% of the outpatient population was sexually compulsive. One would then expect this would be the same or lower for adolescent offenders. Another study on juvenile sexual abusers cited the rate of recidivism in treated offenders to be less than 8% while in untreated offenders it rose to 19%. Although significant, this does suggest that even without treatment more than 80% of juveniles arrested for sexual offenses were not re-arrested in the follow-up period. This contradicts the belief that the majority of adolescent offenders are compelled to sexually abuse others.

Remember also that adolescence is a period of dramatic transition in which sexual maturation is a central component. Changes in the body, brain, and hormones challenge each individual's coping skills. "Practicing," including practicing roles in relationships and becoming familiar with sexual interests, desire, and arousal, is an important developmental task during this period. Adams and Montemayor[5] identify autonomy, intimacy, and sexuality as core components of adolescent development. Erikson[6] noted that sexual behaviors in adolescence are often not driven entirely by a need for sexual gratification. Practicing, seeking acceptance from peers, and buiding self-worth more commonly motivate sexual behaviors.

In O'Brian and Bera's[7] typology of juvenile sex offenders, they refer to one group of offenders as peer influenced: youths who engage in abusive sexual acts to gain peer approval, as in gang activity. There is also a group referred to as "naïve" offenders. These individuals are motivated by their increasing sexual curiosity in adolescence and may also be socially isolated.

SEXUALLY COMPULSIVE ADOLESCENTS: WHO ARE THEY?

The term sexual compulsivity, as discussed in the literature, refers to a broad group of adolescents in which males who commit sexual crimes are but one component and may not be sexually compulsive. As with adults, there is no DSM designation for sexual addiction or compulsive behavior in adolescence. The criteria for adolescents are the same as for adults, although the behaviors may likely be forming rather than established, ingrained patterns of behavior. The criteria for sexual compulsivity is generally thought to include a pattern of out-of-control behaviors; a person risking or suffering consequences as a result of these sexual behaviors; an inability to stop despite the adverse consequences; the use of sexual behavior or fantasy as a primary way of coping; an increasing need to heighten the level of stimulation; inordinate amounts of time spent engaging in sex or seeking sexual encounters; and the neglect of other areas of life such as occupational, academic, recreational, and social activities.

In addition, the same levels of behaviors apply to adolescents as well as adults. Some behaviors may be excessive but socially acceptable, such as masturbation, pornography, and prostitution. Then there are the activities referred to as "nuisance behaviors" that include exhibitionism, voyeurism, and sexual phone calls. Last, there is the level of overtly abusive and dangerous behaviors such as child abuse and sexual assault.

The term sexually compulsive adolescent usually refers to sexually abusive males, but there are those who present clinically who meet all of levels of the behaviors described above. For example, Freeman-Longo[8] refers to the growing number of teens referred for counseling because they use the Internet to seek sexual encounters or visit porn sites. The population of adolescents displaying these behaviors also includes female youths such as adolescent female sexual abusers.[9] Adult female sexual abuse victims often describe having engaged in some sexually abusive behavior in late childhood or adolescence. Beyond this, it has been the author's experience that sexually compulsive behavior frequently emerges within the history of eating disorder patients. Eating disorder behaviors seem to parallel hyper/hypo sexual behaviors. Both include appetite, desire, pleasure/gratification, and satiation. As in the cultural messages about sexuality, the eating disordered patient struggles with issues of "over control" (binging/bulimia) and "under control" (anorexia). Similar behaviors often manifest in hypersexual and hyposexual behaviors with some patients describing periods of aversion to sexual behaviors juxtaposed to periods of "binging" on compulsive, risk-taking sexual behaviors.

DEVELOPMENT OF SEXUALLY COMPULSIVE BEHAVIORS IN ADOLESCENCE

The etiology of sexually compulsive behaviors in adolescence is not different from that of adults, but the patterns emerge at an earlier stage of development. This makes early awareness of behaviors and treatment interventions crucial, so that therapy can halt the sexual compulsivity before the individual suffers from the progressive difficulties that often accompany this disorder. Halting it early may also decrease the transmission of sexually compulsive behaviors to others.

This "transmission to others" refers to childhood sexual abuse or early sexualization as a causative factor in the development of sexual compulsivity and sexually abusive behaviors later in life. Individuals who have been sexually abused are more likely to display a range of psychiatric and emotional problems throughout their life. Eighty-one percent of those persons identified as sexually compulsive report a history of being sexually abused.[10] Sexual abuse, however, is not the only causal factor leading to later sexual addiction.

Studies of sexually abusive male adolescents have identified a combination of factors significant in the development of the abusive behaviors, including chaotic family environment, exposure to domestic violence, exposure to sexually graphic materials, and poor peer relationships.[11,12] Some sexual addicts report no history of childhood sexual abuse but often describe emotional neglect or deficits in the attachment system. Even when sexual abuse has occurred, the context in which it occurs is as important as the event. Insecurely attached children are at higher risk to be abused and have fewer internal as well as external resources to help them cope when abused. Insecurely attached adolescents who have not been sexually abused may turn to sexual behaviors such as excessive masturbation as a way to fill the emotional void or may use sexual behaviors to feel a sense of belonging. Understanding these antecedents is necessary to develop successful treatment interventions. The following discussion will outline the pertinent factors in the treatment of sexually compulsive youth.

TRAUMA, ATTACHMENT, AND SELF-CONCEPT

Psychological trauma generally refers to a situation in which a person is subject to an overwhelming emotional experience that exceeds their ability to understand, accept, and integrate it into their conception of the world. When this "situation" is sexual abuse, the child often has no understanding of adult sexuality and so is exposed to behaviors with no reference point in past experience. As is physiologically expected, the body responds to stimulation and is aroused and, initially, the child may even be gratified by the attention from the perpetrator. The intense and conflicting emotions of confusion, fear, arousal, shame, and anger overload the child's capacity to cope. Unless addressed directly by understanding and caring adults, the child will use some level of dissociation to be able to function.

The severity of dissociation will vary. In some situations, amnesiac barriers remove all awareness of the event. In others, the child may recall the event but detach from the emotional experience. Or the child may dissociate the sensory experience, the touch, pain, smells, and so forth. In any case, what is dissociated is not eliminated; it is encapsulated within the "implicit memory"[13] and remains unintegrated, outside of the person's known narrative. Although this protects the child from being overwhelmed in the moment, the dissociated material retains and freezes the intensity of the experience, so that it will not and cannot decrease over time.

This results in a number of psychological and behavioral symptoms. A bipolar personality may develop around the dissociation, referred to as structural dissociation,[14] in which the child splits into a good me/bad me or day child/night child. In more severe cases, dissociative identity disorder develops in which fragmentation results in multiple identities separated by solid amnesiac barriers that present as distinct personalities with different experiences and traits.

But there are other manifestations of the dissociation. The events that are split off from awareness will intrude into the person's world in some fashion. This is recognized in the criteria for PTSD, which includes flashback, nightmares, and behavioral reenactments. One such behavior is repetition compulsion, the need to reenact aspects of the traumatic event in an unconscious attempt at mastery, to control what was out of control. Specific to sexual addiction, Stoller[15] referred to the reenactment of sexual abuse as "triumph over tragedy," when, in a dissociative state, the individual recreates the sexual experience under the illusion that he or she will master it and thereby resolve it. Within this reenactment is the "victim to victimizer"[16] phenomenon in which the person who was sexually abused seeks a sense of mastery by identifying with the perpetrator. But resolution never occurs through this process. Instead, the person remains compelled to engage in continued sexual behaviors that literally or symbolically recreate the abuse.

When there has been sexual abuse or exposure to sexually graphic or violent acts, the natural unfolding of sexuality is disrupted. Generally, sexual knowledge unfolds via curiosity and self-stimulation in childhood, then on to peer exploration such as mutual masturbation, and later to exploration in early romantic relationships. This natural unfolding is guided by the individual's own interests and takes place within equal relationships, such as between peers who are equal in knowledge and power.

One criterion of sexual abuse is that there is a knowledge and power differential between the victim and abuser. In the abuse, the natural unfolding of sexuality is disrupted by the premature exposure to sexual acts, which may even trigger the early onset of puberty. The abusive sex becomes paired with arousal in a kind of programming that is also encapsulated in dissociated parts of the self. This pairing, or "trauma bond," of sexual arousal to the earlier abuse is a central factor in compulsive reenactment.[17]

While reenactment is central in the consideration of sexually compulsive behavior, it is also imperative to understand the significance of structural dissociation in this process. Marilyn Van Derbur,[18] the former Miss America, describes her experience of being sexually abused in childhood. She relates that there was a split between the "day child" and "night child." Each day she could go to school and excel in academics and other activities, unaware that at night she would await her perpetrator while frozen in a fetal position. This exemplifies what Van der Hart[14] refers to as structural dissociation: the personality is constructed around the traumatic dissociation, and there is the appearance of adequate adjustment or high achievement. But this façade conceals the hidden aspects of the person's life. It is the hidden parts of the self that hold the experience of the abuse and that later engage in the behavioral reenactments. Therefore, it is not uncommon to hear sexually compulsive adolescents as well as adults refer to a double life, a split between what is presented to the world and what is held in the shadow.

A factor related to dissociation is that of objectification. This can refer to both the objectification of the victim or partner (in consensual compulsive sex) as well as an objectification of the sexual compulsive's own body and personhood. A lack of empathy is frequently cited as a trait of sexual abusers. In this, the perpetrator is seen to perceive the victim as a source of gratification and ignore the person's own subjective experience of injury and pain. This is one example of how the "other" is objectified. However, there are other examples of how objectification manifests itself in sexually compulsive behaviors. Individuals have described feeling gratified by a sense of conquest in which the actual sex is of less consequence than the process of seduction—the potential sexual partner is perceived more as prey than lover. In such a description the other's personhood is also ignored, dismissed, and objectified.

Other sexually compulsive individuals have described how they objectify themselves. Eating disorder patients describe a general dissociation from their bodies that also emerges in their sexual behaviors. For example, an adolescent female related how she dissociates and feels removed from her body as she allows her partner to fondle her and then have intercourse. She says she has only disdain for her body and experiences no sensual pleasure. At some level, all sexually compulsive individuals objectify themselves when their compulsive behaviors, motivated by dissociated experiences, separate them from authentic emotion and need.

ATTACHMENT

As noted, not all sexually compulsive individuals have been sexually abused and not all behavioral reenactments are recreations of early sexual abuse. Here, the attachment literature is significant as it seeks to conceptualize other developmental factors in the etiology of sexual compulsions. Attachment theory asserts that one's early infant-caregiver relationships lead to the internalization of self-other mental representations that form the templates for subsequent interpersonal relationships. This includes representations of self in relation to others, which is the basis for one's self-concept. These templates evolve through childhood and adolescence to accommodate the expanded experience of the individual and include the integration of sexuality into one's self-other concept.

The attachment referred to in attachment theory relates to those child/caretaker interactions that revolve around security. Attachment styles are formed by 1 year of age and research has indicated that the style present at 1 year will persist into adulthood. The attachment styles described include: secure, anxious, avoidant, and, more recently delineated, disorganized.

Secure attachment requires an attunement by the caretakers to the child's emotional state and related needs. A secure attachment[19] allows the child the safety from which to explore the world. The ramifications of secure attachment are global. Securely attached children are likely to acknowledge their own emotions and attribute value to their emotions. They have an innate sense of worth and sense of agency. Securely attached children internalize the ability to self soothe.

On the other hand, insecurely attached children do not develop the ability to meet developmental needs in a healthy manner.[20] Low self-esteem, a lack of empathy, poor social skills, and an inability to self soothe are often observed among these children.

Specific to the issue of sexual behaviors are poor self-regulation skills that facilitate withdrawal and acting out. A lack of self-regulation is associated with poor impulse control and increases the incidence of aggressive behaviors. Further, such children will engage in self-stimulating behaviors such as excessive masturbation to escape emotional overload.

Of particular significance to this discussion is the disorganized attachment style, which does not refer to a general psychological confusion but to the absence of a consistent strategy in attachment behaviors. The child is caught between seeking comfort and fearing a hostile response from the parent. Such children may run to a caretaker but then freeze in their steps. Research has associated disorganized attachment with hostile, aggressive behaviors as well as dissociation in children.[21,22]

Given this, one can recognize "attachment trauma" as a critical factor in the development of sexual compulsivity even when sexual abuse is not present.[23] Cyranowski and Anderson[24] contend that it is through the attachment process that one develops sexual self-schemas that guide sexual behaviors.

These schemas evolve through adolescence and change through an interplay of current experience and the internalized models the individual carries from childhood.

SELF-CONCEPT

The prior discussion addresses how the related experiences of attachment, trauma, and dissociation are significant in the development of sexually compulsive behaviors. Woven within this is the evolving self-concept in childhood and adolescence. One way self-concept is affected is by structural dissociation, as mentioned earlier. This occurs when an alternative personality is created to cope with a particular trauma. The person's experience of self is split by a personality that functions, or even achieves, but is dissociated from the traumatic event(s). The person's "emotional self" carries the experience of the trauma. The person will appear to function normally until an environmental or intrapsychic trigger evokes the "emotional self." When this occurs, the person may reexperience the original traumatic event through an overwhelming cascade of emotion, sensory flashback, or behavioral reenactment. Central to this discussion is that the personality is not integrated, leading to a split perception of self, ie, good me/bad me.

Attachment experience also has an impact on the evolving self-concept. Secure attachment is associated with a child attributing value to his or her own subjective experience, developing a sense of agency and worth, and internalizing self-soothing functions. In insecure attachment children are less likely to develop these functions or to attribute value to their own experience. Such individuals lack self-regulation skills and may act out as a way to cope. In the author's own research on the development of sexual aggression, injury to the person's self-concept in childhood and adolescence appeared in the history of perpetrators who were sexually compulsive.

For example, when frequently humiliated or belittled by caretakers, the child perceives that they deserve this treatment. Implicitly, core beliefs about the self develop that reflect the child's experience, such as "I am different," "I am undeserving," "I am defective," and "I am inadequate." Such core beliefs guide self/other interactions but also fuel a shame/rage cycle. In this, an underlying sense of being defective or inadequate evokes shame. But eventually shame will evoke rage that will be acted out against oneself or others. If the source of the shame is based in the child's own sexual abuse it increases the likelihood that the rage will be acted out in sexual behavior.

This is even more likely when the child or adolescent copes with the abuse by identifying with the perpetrator to escape the helplessness and vulnerability of being a victim. The child is thus able to dissociate from the painful experience of the abuse but must take on the identity of the perpetrator and alter his one self-concept: "I am like him" (perpetrator).

In summary, trauma, dissociation, attachment, and self-concept were explored as a precursor to the discussion of treatment interventions for sexually compulsive youth. Before proceeding to the treatment aspect, we conceptualized the underlying factors that influence the overt behaviors. This also impacts the way we perceive sexually compulsive youth, especially those who engage in sexually abusive behaviors. The idea that trauma, dissociation, and attachment injury are consistently present in the histories of sexually compulsive youth raises the dilemma as to whether we characterize these youth as criminals or victims. Based on the conceptualizations discussed here, treatment of the individual's victimization would be central to change but must be balanced against the issues of victimization, accountability, and responsibility.

TREATMENT INTERVENTIONS

Comprehensive treatment requires that a cognitive-behavioral relapse prevention format be included in the treatment of sexually compulsive youth. This begins with an effort to "open the channel" with full disclosure of the abusive or problem behaviors and attempts to remove denial and minimization. The individual seeks to identify the progression of events, thoughts, and emotions that facilitate the problem behaviors. Interventions are designed to impede this pattern. This format would also contain training such as social skills, empathy building, and cognitive restructuring. While these more traditional interventions are necessary, they alone will not effectively redress the trauma, dissociation, and attachment injury.

TRAUMA AND DISSOCIATION

Often when the goal of working on trauma is proposed, the person, particularly if an adolescent, will respond, "I already talked about that" or "I don't need to work on that. It doesn't bother me." Because the trauma has been dissociated, the person may not actually be aware of the impact of the events. Resolution is evident when the person can recount a narrative of the traumatic events without emotional detachment, feeling emotionally overwhelmed, or reliving the event. The goal in treating trauma is to reassociate what has been dissociated, to release trauma bonds, and revise core beliefs formed in the emotional intensity of the traumatic events.

To attain these goals it is necessary to use a model of therapy that can access dissociated experience. This should not be confused with catharsis or spontaneous abreaction, which will not help and can actually reinforce maladaptive reactions and/or be revictimizing. Examples of effective models of therapy include Eye Movement Desensitization Reprocessing (EMDR)[25] and those that provide more direct access, such as Internal Family Systems (IFS) therapy[26] and Ego State Therapy[27] supported with use of the expressive therapies. Both IFS and Ego State Therapy propose that subpersonalities develop within each of us as a way to cope with life circumstances. While this is usually adaptive, problems arise when unacceptable or overwhelming experience is disowned and other subpersonalities develop to manage the conflicting forces within the internal system. An example of this is when the person identifies with the abuser as a way to separate from the disowned part that feels frightened and abused and contains the experience of the abuse.

Both of these therapies allow the client to access and relate to the "parts" of self and the disowned experience. This promotes the resolution of traumatic/dissociative reactions in a number of ways. First, as in the example of identification with the perpetrator, it allows the individual to perceive the internalized perpetrator as a "part" or ego state as opposed to "me." The experience of becoming aware and accessing "parts" facilitates the unblending of the perpetrator part from the self and allows the individual to revise the self-concept.

Second, accessing the disowned experience in this fashion allows the person to re-associate what has been dissociated, be it cognition of the event, or reconnection to the emotional or sensory experience. When this has been integrated into the person's narrative, the intrapsychic pressure no longer intrudes in nightmares, flashbacks, or reenactments. And third, accessing the disowned experience in this manner provides an avenue for the individual to maintain a mature presence but see the events through the child's eyes. The person has a foot in both the present and the past.

Often, distortions formed in the abuse, such as self-blame, are the result of both the child's immaturity (with messages from the abuser) and the person's tendency to view past events through the lens of their present age, stature, and knowledge. For example, an adolescent states, "I should have been able to stop him," or "I shouldn't have let that happen." By accessing the experience of the child, the individual can understand the confusion, fear, and power differential between the perpetrator and the child. This understanding helps to relieve shame, which in turn revises negative perceptions of self, such as "I was at fault," or "I was inadequate."

One critical result of this is compassion for oneself. Here it is important to distinguish between self-compassion and the self-centered, gratification-oriented motivations associated with sexual addicts and sexual abusers. Self-compassion requires an awareness and acceptance of one's authentic emotional experience. Along with this is the motivation to self-soothe in a manner that is not destructive and to treat oneself as deserving. With true self-compassion, one is less likely to objectify oneself or others, thereby decreasing the chances of sexual acting out.

Expressive therapies, used with individual therapy models to access parts of the self, can compliment this process. These may include art, movement, psychodrama, and music therapies. Adolescents, in particular, may be resistant to direct attention to vulnerable parts of self, so art and music can be especially helpful in engaging the individual. Further, the expressive modalities can reinforce insights and connections made in individual sessions. The depiction of past events in art or in psychodrama are both examples of how expressive modalities are used to access dissociated experience.

ATTACHMENT

There are three components in treating the attachment issues of sexually compulsive adolescents. Attachment trauma results from chronic misattunement and neglect; the outcome being an insecure attachment that impacts the adolescent's ego functions, self-concept, and internalized model of relating. In individual therapy this is addressed in much the same fashion as other childhood traumas. Next it is important to address attachment issues through family therapy if possible and, after evaluation, to determine its likely benefit. Skills training in interpersonal effectiveness is also necessary to help the adolescent develop healthy and satisfying relationships.

Individual therapy in treating attachment parallels is what was outlined in the prior section in treating other psychological trauma. Adolescents are often resistant to addressing attachment issues and even more resistant to identifying issues such as trauma. This aversion is partially because of the nature of attachment trauma. Often no singular event stands out as traumatic, but it is the consistent, repetitive nature of the neglect and misattunement to the child's emotional needs that results in maladaptive attachment styles. The absence of a specific traumatic event often leads the individual to minimize the impact. Misplaced loyalties to the family also result in resistance to this work. Perceived and/or direct criticism of parents can trigger the adolescent to feel the need to defend the parent and his or her own distorted interpretations and remembrances of the situation.

As with other types of trauma, minimization serves a defensive function by allowing the individual to avoid the painful emotions related to childhood neglect. It is not uncommon, particularly when working with social services, that an adolescent referred for his or her own sexual behavior problems has also experienced a home environment that includes substance abuse, deprivation, exposure to violence, and graphic sexual behaviors. The adults in such a situation are often literally and/or emotionally absent. The children are left to fend for themselves, which, in addition to the absence of a secure parental presence, makes the child more vulnerable to real-world dangers such as sexual abusers. Working through the denial and minimization is important to help the adolescent recognize what is fact, and to access an authentic emotional response.

To maintain the perception of the "good parents," the adolescent must not only disown the childhood experience of pain and distress, but also redirect the anger that is always generated in neglect. The anger may be disowned, not consciously acknowledged, or manifest itself in a misattribution of blame. In either case it will be misdirected and may be acted out in sexual or other aggressive behaviors. It is also important to understand that attachment trauma and overt and emotional neglect occurs not only in the lower socioeconomic groups, as are often involved with social services, but also in well-educated, financially secure households. Parenting by narcissistic, achievement-oriented, and emotionally closed parents can also result in attachment disorders.

In therapy, this requires the same type of intervention described in the treatment of dissociation and trauma. The adolescent must access the disowned experience and related "parts of self," again with one foot in the experience of the child and the other foot in the present. Also, as was discussed in the treatment of trauma, self-compassion is a necessary goal. Without this, the individual will likely perceive his or her own vulnerability as a weakness, rather than a trait of being human. Males, in particular, are socialized to reject vulnerability as weakness, which then can result in adolescents (and later adults) attacking in others what is disowned in themselves.

Family therapy may be indicated and can have a powerful healing influence, but only if parental figures are available and emotionally viable. As with the sexually compulsive adolescent, the adults must be able to be accountable for their own transgressions and harm to others and can role-model self-responsibility. If the parents are unwilling to be accountable for themselves, or to validate the experience of misattunement and neglect, this could reinforce the defenses of the adolescent. Again, these are the reasons an assessment is necessary before family therapy sessions.

As in individual therapy, family therapy is most effective if there is an emotional component. Family members must to be able to create and hold a space in which the adolescent and adults can be vulnerable. An example of a model of therapy that does focus on attachment issues is Emotionally Focused Therapy (EFT) as developed by Susan Johnson.[28] EFT espouses that "attachment needs and desires and most emotional responses are essentially healthy. How these desires and responses are enacted in the context of perceived danger becomes problematic".[28] Further, Johnson describes emotions as the primary link between self and others and what orients people to their basic needs. Initially developed for marital therapy, others have expanded the use of EFT to treat families.

Insecure attachment is associated with emotional dysregulation. Family members are either reactive or numb. Insecurity influences the processing of information within interpersonal interactions, which often is experienced as others being untrustworthy and/or the self as defective. Therefore, a goal of family therapy sessions is to elicit emotion and guide the interactions so that family members can be direct, honest, and nonabusive. This promotes an environment of safety, validates the authentic emotional experience, and allows the adolescent an avenue to access formally disowned parts of self within interpersonal relationships. The expectation is that this will improve external family relationships and revise the maladaptive internalized models of relating.

Last, in regard to attachment and interpersonal relating, skills training is needed. This would include training in boundaries, communication, and assertiveness, and may also include training in courtship. While a cognitive aspect to this training is necessary, it is also crucial that treatment include an experiential component. Practicing allows the adolescent to develop a sense of familiarity and mastery.

HEALTHY SEXUALITY

To be human is to be a sexual being. Adolescence is when sexuality emerges in a mature form and can be an especially difficult period even within a supportive environment. Several factors can interfere with a person's developing sense of self and relationships with others. Sexually compulsive youth have experienced some combination of these developmental injuries resulting in the use of sex as a way of coping and a seemingly endless cycle of reenactment.

While a disciplined relapse prevention approach is necessary and may help to control the behaviors, merely controlling compelling urges will not restore sexual satisfaction and a sense of worth. After a person has attained a period of abstinence and worked through injuries as outlined in this paper, it is then necessary to help the person develop a healthy sexuality. Price[29] calls for a treatment model based on developing a healthy sexuality and that carefully considers the developmental tasks of adolescence. The risks of not addressing this, according to Price, is that simply removing the "deviant" arousal leaves a vacuum that might be filled by a regression to the deviant if a healthy sexuality is not available to replace it. Price notes that an adolescent who remains conflicted or confused about sexuality is likely to maintain a negative self-concept and feel unaccepted by others.

A format to develop healthy sexuality would include sex education (reproduction and anatomy); relationship skills training as described earlier; and an exploration of one's own sexual orientation, gender identity, sexual values/morality and intimacy. This is of particular significance when one's arousal is trauma bonded to a past injury. In such a situation individuals often consider the reenactment as their sexual identity, ie, sado-masochism, sexually aggressive, dangerous, or risk-taking behaviors. While the psychotherapy described earlier is designed to release the person from the trauma bond, adolescents are often left with confusion as to what is healthy sexuality.

Exploration and clarification is then needed to develop a sexual identity that is acceptable and authentic. This is difficult in that there is no consensus as to what criteria define healthy sexuality. To address this dilemma, Price[29] referred to developmental theorists such as Erickson,[6] Bandura,[30] and Kohlberg[31] to identify the developmental tasks of adolescence and used this as a guide to target goals and necessary skills. When addressing issues of sexual orientation, however, the sexual attitudes, values, and beliefs of the clinical staff and society will influence the adolescent in treatment.

As in other aspects of treatment, the individual must attain a sense of identity that is honest and accepted by those around them. Therefore, the clinical staff will need to help each youth clarify what is authentic for him or her. To help with this, the treatment of eating disorders offers a beneficial parallel. The anorexic, over time loses awareness of natural functions and cues such as appetite, hunger/fullness, gratification, and satiation. The behavior is rewarded, however, by the sense of identity and achievement that results from the self-deprivation (trauma bond). Treatment is guided by the idea that the patient does not need to create something that is not there but to be mindful and restore awareness of natural functions. In the same way (after releasing the trauma-bonded sexual urges), the sexually compulsive adolescent can be helped to become aware of authentic responses such as attraction, desire, arousal, emotions, and their related needs. With compassionate guidance and helping the adolescent to feel accepted by others, the individual will eventually learn how to know and accept him- or herself.

SUMMARY

We clarified the nature of sexual compulsivity in adolescence, addressed who is labeled as "sexually compulsive youth," conceptualized the underlying factors of sexual compulsivity, and outlined a treatment format. We focused on trauma, dissociation, attachment, and self-concept. We questioned the conventional perceptions of who is included in this group. We reiterated that the belief that sexually compulsive adolescents are abusive males is no longer considered accurate. The evolution and accessibility of the Internet only raises greater concerns about compulsive sexual behavior, as more adolescents are brought into therapy because of Internet use to seek sexual interaction or stimulation. The sexually compulsive youth is as likely to be the clean-cut, high-achieving, intelligent student as is the economically deprived, juvenile delinquent on the street.

This article began with the observation that adolescents rarely receive any direct, accurate information about sexuality and intimacy. The messages taken in through music, television, movies, politicians, popular press, clergy, and school are polarizing and contradictory. Beyond this are the implications as to how we, as a society, treat the youths that do present with sexual behavior problems. We have tended to treat these youth (as well as adults) with disdain and to designate sexually abusive youth the same as adult offenders with harsher, more punitive treatment interventions. Research and clinical experience now strongly question this type of response.

This article is consistent with this leaning. Early psychological injury, from sexual abuse, physical abuse, exposure to violence, attachment trauma, or early sexualization, is at the root of sexually compulsive behavior. While it is necessary to reign in out-of-control and destructive behaviors, if we acknowledge that the source of the behavior is psychological injury, then it is cruel and inconsistent to treat the individual with disdain or as a pariah. The same dilemma is present with adult sexual addicts and offenders. Our society must develop a response to sexually compulsive or offensive behavior that can protect those who need protection, while implementing a rational legal response and providing treatment options for the underlying injury. Perhaps even more importantly, our society must learn how to educate adolescents about sexuality with clear, accurate information that includes not only reproduction but sexual response and intimacy as well.

REFERENCES

1. Hirsch B. A comparison of normal sexual development and sexual abuse in children. Critique and recommendations for training [doctoral dissertation]. The California School of Professional Psychology. California 1999.
2. Money J. Principles of developmental sexology. New York: Continuum; 1997.
3. Letourneau EJ. Juvenile sex offenders: a case against the status quo. Sexual Abuse 2005;17(3):293–312.
4. Marshall WL, Marshall LE. Sexual addiction among incarcerated sexual offenders. Sexual Addiction and Compulsivity 2006;13(4):377–90.
5. Adams GR, Montemayor R. Psychosocial development during adolescence. California (CA): Sage Publications; 1996.
6. Erickson EH. Identity: youth and crisis. New York: Norton; 1968.
7. O'Brian M, Bera W. Adolescent sexual offenders: a descriptive typology. Newsletter of the Family Life Education Network 1986;5:22–5.
8. Freeman-Longo RE. Children, teens and sex on the Internet. Sexual Addiction and Compulsivity 2000;7:75–90.
9. Bumby KM, Halstenson Bumby N. Adolescent female adolescent offenders. In: Schwartz B, Cellini HR, editors. The sex offender: new insights, treatment innovations and legal developments. New Jersey (NJ): Civic Research Institute; 1997. p. 10-11 –10-15.
10. Carnes P. The obsessive shadow: profiles in sexual addiction. Professional Counselor 1998;13(1):15–7, 40–41.
11. Borduin C, Blaske D. Individual, family and peer characteristics of adolescent sex offenders and assaultive offenders. Dev Psychol 1989;25(5):86–99.
12. Oster M. An examination of family dynamics contributing to intrafamily sexual offending by male adolescents [doctoral dissertation]. California School of Professional Psychology. San Diego 1999.
13. Van der Kolk B. The body keeps the score: memory and the evolving psychobiology of potsttraumatic stress. Harv Rev Psychiatry 1994;1:253–65.
14. Van der Hart O, Nijenhuis E, Steele K. The haunted self: structural dissociation and the treatment of chronic traumatization. New York: W.W. Norton & Cie; 2006.
15. Stoller R. Perversion: the erotic form of hatred. New York: Pantheon Books; 1975.
16. Schwartz M. In my opinion: victim to victimizer. Sexual Addiction and Compulsivity 1995;2(2):81–8.
17. Schwartz M. Reenactments related to bonding and hypersexuality. Sexual Addiction and Compulsivity 1996;3(3):195–211.
18. Van Derbur M. Miss America by day: lessons learned from ultimate betrayal and unconditional love. Denver (CO): Oak Hill Press; 2004.
19. Bowlby J. The making and breaking of affectional bonds. London: Routledge; 1979.
20. Lyons-Ruth K. Attachment relationships among children with aggressive behavior problems: the role of disorganized attachment patterns. J Consult Clin Psychol 1996;64(1):64–73.
21. Alpern L, Lyons-Ruth K. Disorganized attachment classification and maternal psychosocial problems as predictors of aggressive behaviors in preschool children. Child Dev 1996;64(2):572–85.

22. Cicchetti D, Toth SL. Child maltreatment and attachment organization. In: Goldberg S, Muir R, Kerr J, editors. Attachment theory: social, developmental and clinical perspectives. Hillsdale (NJ): The Analytic Press; 1995.
23. Cooper ML, Shapiro CM, Powers AM. Motivations for sex and risky sexual behaviors among adolescents and young adults: a functional perspective. J Pers Soc Psychol 1998;75(6):1528–58.
24. Cyranowski JM, Andersen BL. Schemas, sexuality and romantic attachment. J Pers Soc Psychol 1998;74(5):1364–79.
25. Shapiro F. Efficacy of eye movement desensitization procedure in the treatment of traumatic memories. J Trauma Stress 1989;2:199–223.
26. Schwartz R. Internal family systems therapy. New York: Guilford Press; 1995.
27. Watkins J, Watkins H. Ego states: theory and therapy. New York: Norton; 1997.
28. Johnson S. The practice of emotionally focused therapy: creating connection. New York: Brunner/Mazel; 1996.
29. Price D. Developmental perspective of treatment for sexually vulnerable youth. Sexual Addiction and Compulsivity 2003;10(4):225–45.
30. Bandura A. Social learning theory. New Jersey (NJ): Prentice-Hall; 1977.
31. Kohlberg L. The psychology of moral development: nature and validity of moral stages. San Francisco: Harper & Row; 1984.

Pharmacology of Sexually Compulsive Behavior

Victoria L. Codispoti, MD, D-FAPA

KEYWORDS

- Pharmacology • Cyproterone acetate
- Medroxyprogesterone acetate • LHRH • Paraphilias
- Selective serotonin reuptake inhibitors (SSRI's)

The history of pharmacological treatment of compulsive sexual behaviors, which are now commonly categorized as paraphilic and non-paraphilic behaviors, has been long and controversial. This article discusses treatments of paraphilic behavior, focusing particularly on sex offenders.

Sexual behavior is the fulfillment of a basic human desire, much like eating is the fulfillment of the basic drive of hunger. If the drive is abnormal, its fulfillment can also be abnormal (as in the case of aberrant sexuality). The biologic precursors to sexual drive are hormones and transmitters,[1] and therefore treatment of deviant sexuality or hypersexuality should include hormonal agents (antiandrogens) and psychotropics (which affect neurotransmitters).

Testosterone strongly influences sexual behavior, particularly in men, and its effects are the basis for hormonal treatment. Decreased levels of serotonin and dopamine also produce decreased sexual drive. Conversely, high levels of these neurotransmitters increase sexual drive. Beyond this knowledge, the role of serotonin is complex and much remains unknown about its operation; additional research into this area is essential.

Management of deviant sexuality through pharmacologic treatment of hypersexuality originated in the 1940s for controlling sex crimes. At that time, courts sometimes ordered surgical castration (removal of the testes) for sex offenders. This method soon proved ineffective, however, because although castration lowers circulating levels of testosterone and diminishes sexual drive, it does not completely eliminate sexual functioning. In a postcastration study of approximately 103 men in Germany,[2] more than 75% of men experienced extinction of libido and sexual activity within 6 months, 15% of men retained some libido and could engage in sexual activity with intense stimulation, and the remaining 10% reported only reduced libido and

Private Practice, #6 Salem Business Center South, Salem, IL 62853, USA

E-mail address: lcodis2000@aol.com

Psychiatr Clin N Am 31 (2008) 671–679
doi:10.1016/j.psc.2008.06.002
0193-953X/08/$ – see front matter. Published by Elsevier Inc.

psych.theclinics.com

sexual activity. Many adverse side effects were produced as a consequence of the surgery, such as decreased protein levels, changes in fat distribution, decreased bone calcium, hot flashes, and decreased body and facial hair. Castration eventually fell out of favor, but its ineffectiveness and the legal system's entree into the field of hypersexual behavior helped spur research into causes and treatments of sexual disorders in hopes of reducing recidivism rates of criminal sexual behavior.

In 1958, Dr. John Money[3,4] of Johns Hopkins University Hospitals completed the first successful pharmacologic treatment of deviant sexual behavior using medroxyprogesterone acetate (MPA) to inhibit libido in those experiencing nonparaphilic hypersexuality and in sex offenders. The drug decreased sexual drive and urges. At that time, estrogens and psychiatric medications, such as tricyclic antidepressants and lithium, were being used without benefit.[5] In the 1960s, psychiatrists began to use MPA with their patients. Cyproterone acetate (CPA), a similar drug that is not available in the United States, was used in Canada and Europe.

PARAPHILIAS AS A SPECTRUM DISORDER

The *Diagnostic and Statistical Manual of Mental Disorders, Fourth Edition, Text Revision* (DSM IV-TR) defines paraphilia as a disorder characterized by recurrent, intense, sexually arousing fantasies and urges, or behaviors generally involving nonhuman objects, suffering or humiliation of one's self or partner, or children or nonconsenting partners. These behaviors must occur over a period of at least 6 months. In some cases, paraphilia preferences occur only episodically (possibly secondary to anxiety), and at other times are necessary for sexual functioning. To be diagnosed as having a paraphilia, the urges or behaviors must cause significant stress or impaired functioning, either occupationally or socially.[6]

Pedophilia is a specific biologic drive involving an erotic and sexual attraction to children or adolescents. A pedophiliac sexual orientation is extremely difficult, if not impossible, to alter. Some pedophiles fantasize frequently when seeing their desired "love" object but do not offend. Others do not fantasize as often, but because of problematic core issues (eg, attachment disorders or a past history of sexual abuse) will develop abnormal relationships with children that culminate in sexual behavior. For others who offend against children, issues of power are more causative. Pedophiles have severe difficulty cognitively comprehending that their feelings and behaviors are abusive or abnormal.

Over the past 15 years, the paraphilia-as-obsessive-compulsive-spectrum-disorder paradigm has met with increasing acceptance. Sexually deviant fantasies are frequently obsessive and will not remit.[6] Paraphilic urges are compulsive and accompanied by anxiety. When urges are acted on, anxiety decreases but the fantasies soon return. The DSM IV-TR defines obsessions as "persistent urges, thoughts, impulses or images that are experienced as intrusive and inappropriate and cause marked anxiety or distress".[7] Obsessions are ego-dystonic (ie, "alien" to the person and not the kinds of thoughts someone would expect to have). Compulsions are repetitive behaviors or mental acts used to reduce anxiety rather than provide pleasure or gratification.

Some individuals who have paraphilias can often have normative sex without the disorder interfering. Others must fantasize about objects or humiliation to function sexually and be orgasmic. Not all individuals who have paraphilias commit crimes. Some say they derive no sexual pleasure from their behavior but merely a release of anxiety. They enter treatment because their lives are severely affected by their sexual compulsions and preferences or their behaviors are illegal and they are court ordered to undergo treatment that may include psychopharmacologic medication to reduce recidivism.

In 1997, the Supreme Court upheld the *Kansas v. Hendricks*[8] decision as constitutional, which meant that sexually violent predators could be civilly committed for treatment. Sexual offenders could be placed in psychiatric hospitals or other treatment facilities after incarceration but before release. In addition to cognitive–behavioral therapy, some individuals also undergo pharmacologic treatment before release into the community. Truthfulness and compliance are essential aspects of treatment and help determine drug dosing levels and length of treatment.

PHARMACOLOGIC TREATMENT

Sex offenders who have severe obsessive fantasies will frequently act on them. McConaghy[9] theorized that sex offenders' inability to refrain is impaired because their general arousal system (as opposed to simply their sexual system) is highly activated, secondary to deficiencies in 5-HT, oxytocin, and vasopressin. Low levels of these transmitters increase testosterone and result in increased sexual drive, aggressiveness, and irritability. Once a behavior is performed, it activates a particular part of the brain. If the urge is not performed in subsequent arousals, tension and excitement increase. This dynamic causes individuals to lose control and continue inappropriate sexual behavior despite known consequences, as if they are addicted.

Implicated in this is the dopaminergic transmission in the limbic forebrain where behaviors associated with attachment are encoded[10] and dysregulation of vasopressin, oxytocin, norepinephrine, and endogenous opioids is found.[11] Currently, evidence shows that pharmacologic treatment targeting these systems is effective for sexual offenders. Medications have been shown to decrease the intensity and frequency of fantasies, the frequency of erections, sexually deviant urges, and anxiety (resulting in a calming effect). No strong evidence shows, however, that recidivism is decreased, because too few well-controlled blinded trials with sufficient sample sizes have been conducted. This article provides a more detailed look at specific chemical interventions.[12,13]

Selective Serotonin Reuptake Inhibitors

Selective serotonin reuptake inhibitors (SSRIs) are used primarily to treat depression, phobia, anxiety, and obsessive compulsive disorder. Numerous studies have also shown SSRIs to be promising in the treatment of sexually compulsive behaviors. Because low or high serotonin levels affect sexual behavior and desire, SSRIs are useful in that they affect both pre- and postsynaptic serotonergic neurons involving numerous subgroups of the 5-HT receptors. More research is needed to determine which subtypes control specific behaviors.[14,15]

Examinations of structural brain abnormalities in patients who have neurologic illnesses, such as epilepsy or Tourette's syndrome, have shown serotonin-related neurocircuitry that may contribute to the pathophysiology of pedophilia. Researchers using voxel-based morphometry[16] have found reduced brain volume in several interconnected areas of the frontostriatal brain, including a neurophysiologic circuit formed by the orbitofrontal cortex and putamen. These anatomic areas belong to the serotonergic system, and have been linked to obsessive–compulsive spectrum disorders in studies of 5-HT dysregulation and second messenger disturbances.[11,17]

Neurons containing 5-HT send axons throughout the brain, including the limbic system and neocortex, affecting levels of oxytocin and vasopressin. Treatment with SSRIs seems to mediate the obsessive–compulsive nature of the sexual fantasies, thereby decreasing their frequency and intensity, and general sexual appetitive behavior. Paraphilics who have chronic life stressors, such as a history of physical or sexual abuse, neglect, abandonment, divorce, also have increased corticotrophin-releasing factor. These changes are associated with hypocampal atrophy and abnormal levels of oxytocin and vasopressin. The SSRI fluoxetine has been shown effective in improving mood and reducing inappropriate sexual behavior in paraphilics and sex addicts, which can be accomplished with an average daily dosing of 40 mg.[15]

In 1994, Kafka reported the results of using sertraline in an open trial with men suffering from paraphilia or paraphilia-related disorders. After 18 weeks, there was significant reduction in the variety of unconventional sexual outlets as well as the frequency of behaviors in both types of subjects. These effects were independent of baseline depression scores. Men for whom treatment with sertraline failed were given fluoxetine, with clinically significant effects.[16]

A 12-week open-label, dose-titration study using sertraline with adult male pedophiles in outpatient treatment resulted in statistically significant improvements. This SSRI decreased urges toward young girls, sexual activity, penile tumescence to audiotape, obsessions, and masturbation. The study concluded that sertraline is well tolerated and effective in treating pedophiles.[17]

Because antiandrogens can cause depression, SSRIs are often used effectively in conjunction with antiandrogens to ease this side effect. The question remains whether the depression is caused by the individual's loss of sexual fantasies, desire, and behaviors, or is a physiologic effect of the antiandrogens.[18]

Medroxyprogesterone Acetate

MPA is a progestational agent that reduces testosterone 5α reductase in the liver, which increases clearance and decreases testosterone levels in serum and tissues and decreases gonadotropin secretion. MPA is not a true antiandrogen, because it does not compete with the androgen receptors. Side effects include decreased spermatogenesis, weight gain, deep vein thrombosis, osteoporosis, soreness, gynecomastia, hot flashes, nausea, vomiting, and soreness at the injection site. Reductions in sex drive, sexual fantasy, and sexual activity are frequently observed. In the laboratory setting, significant reduction in arousal to erotic stimuli was statistically significant, with reduced nocturnal penile tumescence.[19]

The best candidates for treatment with MPA are those who admit to their offenses, experience compelling sexual fantasies that they report as causing confusion and poor cognitive functioning, and who have overwhelming and uncontrollable compulsions. Some patients have reported that MPA reduces "the noise level" in their head (referring to the constant intrusion of sexual fantasies), and allows them to think more clearly and gain more benefit from therapy than without the medication.

MPA was used initially in open trials to treat nine paraphilic men at a dose of 300 to 400 mg intramuscularly each week. Positive treatment response was observed continuously for up to 8 years later in some subjects. Two separate open clinical studies of 20 paraphilic men and 48 patients[20] showed that MPA was effective if patients were compliant. Discontinuation of medications resulted in a significant relapse rate.

MPA can be used intramuscularly to ensure compliance at doses from 200 to 600 mg weekly, biweekly, or monthly. Sexual response must be measured to titrate the dosage. Oral MPA can be made available if the individual's compliance is assured.

Cyproterone Acetate

Testosterone is the most significant androgen influencing male sexual behavior. CPA (not available in the United States) is a powerful antiandrogen and antigonadotropic.

Its specific mode of action is competitive inhibition of testosterone and dihydrotesterone at the androgen receptor.

CPA is the most widely studied pharmacologic agent for treating the paraphilias. A study of 100 men in Germany,[21] including pedophiles, sadists, and exhibitionists, showed that men given 100 mg of CPA once daily experienced decreased sex drive, reduced erections, and fewer orgasms. Lower doses reduced libido but allowed erections and some sexual behaviors.

Side effects are similar to those of MPA, but also include liver dysfunction, adrenal suppression, osteoporosis, fatigue, varicose veins, and hair loss.

Contraindications for its use are a history of thromboembolism, renal failure, liver disease, protein malnutrition, and cancer chemotherapy.

Numerous studies have shown CPA to be effective in reducing deviant sexual behavior, including large studies of up to 200 patients. Duration of treatments varied from 2 months to 8 years. Dosages ranged from 50 to 100 mg orally to 300 to 600 mg intramuscularly weekly or biweekly. Results showed reduced libido, decreased nocturnal penile tumescence, reduced paraphilic fantasies, and a reduction in paraphilic behavior.[22] A double-blind placebo crossover study of CPA in 19 men concluded that the drug was associated with a significant reduction of sexual fantasies. The study also suggests that CPA is not indicated for sexual behavior that is not sexually driven or paraphilic.[23]

In a study on pedophilic sexual arousal patterns,[24] subjects were divided into high and low testosterone groups. CPA seemed to have a differential response on the groups; it was more effective at reducing deviant sexual arousal to pedophilic stimuli than reducing arousal to nondeviant sex. This finding could be interpreted as "normalizing" the sexual arousal patterns of pedophiles.

CPA as a pharmacologic agent for paraphilia has been extensively studied with regard to treatment outcomes and recidivism. Several studies have shown it to be effective in significantly reducing posttreatment recidivism rates during 1- to 5-year follow-up periods.[24,25,26]

LUTEINIZING HORMONE–RELEASING HORMONE

Luteinizing hormone–releasing hormone (LHRH) is synthesized in the cell bodies of the hypothalamic nuclei and stimulates gonadotropic cells to release gonadotropin-releasing hormone (GnRH) and follicle-stimulating hormone (FSH). These hormones then stimulate gonadal production of sex steroids. Continuous application of a long-acting LHRH agonist suppresses the pituitary–gonadal axis. Secretion of FSH and LH is inhibited and testosterone drops to castration levels. Leuprolide acetate is a long-acting analog GnRH that inhibits production of testosterone through overwhelming the feedback loop. Urologists often use leuprolide to treat prostatic cancer because of its effectiveness in decreasing testosterone. Leuprolide decreases sexual desire, fantasies, and urges, and significantly decreases the frequency of masturbation.[27,28]

Injection of the shorter-acting LHRH to treat pedophilia shows a greater increase in LH but not FSH. Pedophilic interest, unfortunately, can be controlled, but not eliminated, because it is a sexual drive aimed at children. Some pedophiles given LHRH could still generate clinically significant penile blood flow in response to children.

Studies of leuprolide acetate have noted similar results for decreasing testosterone and its consequences. Additional positive responses are decreased distractibility and improvement in cognitive function and comprehension. Individuals' ability to recognize triggers for behaviors was greatly improved because they were not distracted by their obsessive–compulsive thoughts. These improvements can be significant in helping individuals derive greater benefit from treatment.

Case reports showed that leuprolide acetate decreased sexual fantasies in one subject prone to exhibitionism, and provided a successful treatment in a homosexual pedophile. One report of a patient who had multiple paraphilias and was resistant to treatment (CPA and MPA) reported marked improvement in fantasies and behaviors while undergoing treatment with leuprolide acetate.

Thibault and colleagues[29] used an LHRH agonist in six patients who had paraphilias, showing good response that ended when the medication was withdrawn. Another study of 30 men treated from 8 to 42 months[30] with psychotherapy and leuprolide showed a reduction in deviant sexual behavior and diminished fantasies. Schober reports that the drug was effective in controlling pedophilic urges during a 2-year period of a blinded study. Two individuals who were in the blinded group expressed great distress that they might offend, and asked to receive the medication.

Dosing of leuprolide is usually 7.5 or 22.5 mg injected intramuscularly once every 3 months, or more frequently if necessary. Side effects are the same as treatment with CPA, which is also an LHRH inhibitor that antagonizes the action of testosterone.

Triptoreline is another agonist analog of GnRH given in monthly injections of 3.75 mg. Rosler and Wetzum's[31] triptoreline study of 40 men resulted in 24 who reported a decrease in the number of their deviant sexual fantasies, desires, and abnormal sexual behaviors while on the drug for at least 1 year.

Other Treatments

Two single case reports showed improvement in paraphilic behavior with topiramate, naltrexone, and monoamine oxidase inhibitors. The patient receiving naltrexone was also diagnosed with kleptomania and paraphilic compulsive sexual behavior, driven by stress. His compulsive sexual behavior included an insatiable need for sequential multiple sexual partners.

At an eventual dose of 150 mg/d of naltrexone, this patient could walk into a store (a previous trigger for his kleptomania) without urges to steal. He then noted that he was sexual with his wife and had no urges to seek other partners.[32]

In another case, topiramate was reported to improve compulsive sexual behavior. This response was believed to be caused by its action on the brain pathways that underlie conditioned behaviors associated with environmental cues. This mechanism would also explain its effectiveness in treating intrusive thoughts and nightmares seen in the posttraumatic stress disorder (PTSD) of incest survivors, triggered by environmental cures.

Kafka[33] hypothesizes that monoamine oxidase transmitters, such as norepinephrine, dopamine, and serotonin, can facilitate and inhibit biologic drives and appetitive behavior. He notes that some paraphilic disorders seem to have axis I comorbid associations and nonsexual psychopathologies that are also associated with monoaminergic dysregulation. However, it is too early to conclude whether these modulators are important in the pathophysiology of paraphilic and sexual aggression.

ATTACHMENT DISORDER THEORY

Studies on attachment disorders describe insecure attachment styles arising from dysfunctional childhood relationships. If these disorders affect brain chemistry and function (as studies report), then offenders from these backgrounds will ultimately form inappropriate or aggressive attachments with adult women, men, or children.[34]

Highly traumatic childhood experiences can result in corticosteroid abnormalities that persist into adulthood and can interact with oxytocin and vasopressin systems. These changes are believed to correlate with attachment deficits.[35,36] The corticosteroids are dependent on 5-HT, which has been shown in animal studies to improve social grooming and cohesiveness, and to increase sexual appetite.

Pearson[37] and Kafka and Coleman[38] have suggested that problems in 5-HT transmission to the dorse raphe nucleus in the brain underlie paraphilic/compulsive disorders and deviant sexual behaviors. These theories are exciting in that they might begin to explain the biophysiologic development of numerous psychiatric disorders. Reviewing the physiologic correlates of compulsive sexual behavior and PTSD brings to mind the concept of a behavior triggered by an environmental cue that is then reflexively acted on without the ability to control it, as is often seen in victims of combat or sexual abuse.

SUMMARY

In a meta-analysis on controlled outcomes evaluations of 22,000 sex offenders, Losel and Schmucker[39] found 80 comparisons between treatment and control groups. The recidivism rate averaged 19% in treated groups, and 27% in controls. Most other reviews reported a lower rate of sexual recidivism in treated sexual offenders.

Of 2039 citations in this study (including literature in five languages), 60 studies held independent comparisons. Problematic issues included the control groups; various hormonal, surgical, cognitive behavioral, and psychotherapeutic treatments; and sample sizes.

In the 80 studies compared after the year 2000, 32% were reported after 2000, 45% originated in the United States, 45% were reported in journals, and 36% were unpublished. Treatment characteristics showed a significant lack of pharmacologic treatment (7.5%), whereas use cognitive and classical behavioral therapy was 64%. In 68% of the studies, no information was available on the integrity of the treatment implementation; 36% of the treatment settings were outpatient only, 31% were prison settings, and 12% were mixed settings (prison, hospital, and outpatient).

Integrating research interpretations is complicated by the heterogeneity of sex offenders, with only 56% being adult men and 17.5% adolescents. Offense types reported included 74% child molestation, 48% incest, and 30% exhibitionism. Pedophilia was not singled out. Follow-up periods varied from 12 months to greater than 84 months. The definition of recidivism ran the gamut from arrest (24%), conviction (30%), charges (19%), and no indication (16%).

Results were difficult to interpret because of the methodological problems with this type of study. Overall, a positive outcome was noted with sex offender treatment. Cognitive–behavioral and hormonal treatment were the most promising. Voluntary treatment led to a slightly better outcome than mandatory participation. When accounting for a low base rate of sexual recidivism, the reduction was 37%, which included psychological and medical modes of treatment.

Which treatments will reduce recidivism rates in sex offenders is extremely difficult to conclude. Some treatment effects are determined from small studies; however, recidivism rates may be based on different criteria. Larger studies tend to be published more frequently than small studies, negative results may be less likely to be reported in published studies, and differences in mandatory versus voluntary treatment may occur.

Clearly more high-quality outcome studies are needed to determine which treatments work best for which individuals. One size is unlikely to fit all. However, pharmacologic intervention, although not always the perfect choice, has improved and will continue to advance the treatment of paraphilic, nonparaphilic, and compulsive sexual behaviors.

REFERENCES

1. Bancroft J. The biological basis of human sexuality. In: Human sexuality and its problems. Edinburgh (Scotland): Churchill Livingstone; 1989. p. 12–127.
2. Wille R, Beier KM. Castration in Germany. Annals of Sex Research 1989;2. p. 103, 107.
3. Money J. Discussion of hormonal inhibition of libido in male sex offenders. In: Michael R, editor. Endocrinology and human behavior. London: Oxford University Press; 1968. p. 169.
4. Money J. Use of androgen-depleting hormone in the treatment of male sex offenders. J Sex Res 1970;6:165–72.
5. Hill A, Briken P, Kraus C, et al. Differential pharmacological treatment of paraphilias and sex offenders. Int J Offender Ther Comp Criminol 2003;47:407.
6. American Psychiatric Association. Diagnostic and statistical manual of mental disorders. 4th edition, [text revision]. Washington, DC: American Psychiatric Press; 2000. 355–6.
7. Bradford JM. Medical interventions in sexual deviance. In: Laws DR, O'Donahue W, editors. Sexual deviance: theory, assessment, and treatment. New York: Guilford Press; 1997. p. 449–64.
8. Kansas v. Hendricks, 521 U.S. 346 (1997).
9. McConaghy N. Sexual behavior: problems and management. New York: Plenum Press; 1993.
10. Bradford JMW. Pharmacological treatment of the paraphilias. In: Oldham JM, Riba M, editors, Review of psych, vol. 14. Washington, DC: American Psychiatric Press; 1995. p. 755–78.
11. Bradford JMW. The treatment of sexual deviation using a pharmacological approach. J Sex Res August 2000.
12. Schiffer B, Peschel T, Paul T. Structural brain abnormalities in the frontostriatal system and cerebellum in pedophilia. J Psychiatr Res 2007;41(9):753–62.
13. Bremner JD, Licinio J, Darnell A, et al. Elevated corticotrophin-releasing factor concentrations in posttraumatic stress disorder. Am J Psychiatry 1997;624–9.
14. Baumgarten HG, Grozdanovic Z. Psychopharmacology of central serotonergic Systems. Pharmacopsychiatry 1995;28(Suppl 2):73–9.
15. Kafka MP, Prentky R. Fluoxetine treatment of non-paraphilic sexual addictions and paraphilias in men. J Clin Psychiatry 1992;53:351–8.
16. Kafka KM. Sertraline pharmacotherapy for paraphilias and paraphilia-related disorders: an open trial. Ann Clin Psychiatry 1994;6:189–95.
17. Bradford JMW, Marlindale JJ, Lane R, et al. Sertraline in the treatment of paraphilia: an open label study. Submitted for publication.
18. Berlin FS, Meinecke CF. Treatment of sex offenders with anti-androgenic medication: conceptualization, review of treatment modalities and preliminary findings. Am J Psychiatry 1981;138:601–7.
19. Wincze WP, Bansal S, Malamud M. Effects of medroxyprogesterone acetate on subjective arousal, arousal to erotic stimulation and nocturnal penile tumescence in male sex offenders. Arch Sex Behav 1986;15:203–305.
20. Gagne P. Treatment of sex offenders with medroxyprogesterone acetate. Am J Psychiatry 1981;138:644–6.
21. Laschet V, Laschet L. Psychopharmacotherapy in sex offenders with cytoproterone acetate. Neuro-Pharmakopsychiatrie 2001;4:99–104.
22. Laschet V, Laschet L. Antiandrogens in the treatment of sexual deviations of men. Journal of Steroid Biochemistry 1975;6:821–6.

23. Bradford JMW, Pawlak MA. Double-blind placebo crossover study of CPA in treatment of the paraphilias. Arch Sex Behav 1993;22:383–402.
24. Bradford JMW, Pawlak MA. Effects of cyproterone acetate on sexual arousal patterns of pedophiles. Arch Sex Behav 1993;22:629–41.
25. Cooper AJ, Ismail AA, Phanjoo AL, et al. Antiandrogen (cytoproterone acetate) therapy in deviant hypersexuality. Br J Psychiatry 1972;120:59–63.
26. Cooper AJ. A placebo controlled study of anti-androgen cyproterone acetate in deviant hypersexuality. Compr Psychiatry 1981;22:458–64.
27. Briken P, Nika E, Berner W. Treatment of paraphilias with LHRH agonists. J Sex Marital Ther 2001;27:45–55.
28. Schober JM, Kuhn PJ, Kovacs P, et al. Leuprolide acetate suppresses pedophilic urges and arousability. Arch Sex Behav 2005;34:691–705.
29. Schober JM, Byrne PM, Kuhn PJ. Leuprolide acetate is a familiar drug that may modify sex-offender behavior: the urologist's role. BJU Int 2006;97:684–6.
30. Thibault E, Cordier B, Kuhn JM. Effect of a long-lasting gonadotrophin hormone-releasing hormone agonist in six cases of severe male paraphilia. Acta Psychiatr Scand 1993;87:445–50.
31. Rosler A, Wetzum E. Treatment of men with paraphilia with a long acting analogue of gonadotropin releasing hormone. N Engl J Med 1998;338:416–22.
32. Grant JE, Kim SW. A case of kleptomania and compulsive sexual behavior treated with naltrexone. American Academy of Clinical Psychology 2002;229–31.
33. Kafka M. The monoamine hypothesis for the pathophysiology of paraphilic disorders: an update. Ann N Y Acad Sci 2003;989(1):86–9.
34. Carter CS. Neuroendocrine perspectives on social attachment and love. Psychoneuroendocrinology 1998;23:779–818.
35. Nelson EE, Panskepp J. Brain substrates of infant-mother-attachment, contributions of opioids, oxytocin, and noroepinephrine. Neurosci Biobehav Rev 1998;22. 437–52.
36. Beech AR, Mitchell IJ. A neurobiological perspective on attachment problems in sexual offenders and the role of selective serotonin re-uptake inhibitors in the treatment of such problems. Clin Psychol Rev 2005;25:153–82.
37. Pearson HJ. Paraphilias, impulse control, and serotonin. J Clin Psychopharmacol 1990;10:233.
38. Kafka MP, Coleman E. Serotonin and paraphilias: the convergence of mood, impulse and compulsive disorders. J Clin Psychopharmacol 1991;223–4.
39. Losel F, Schmucker M. The effectiveness of treatment for sexual offenders: a comprehensive meta-analysis. J Exper Crim 2005;1:117–46.

Sexual Offender Treatment: a Positive Approach

William L. Marshall, OC, PhD, FRSC[a,b,*], Liam E. Marshall, MA[a],
Gerris A. Serran, PhD[a], Matt D. O'Brien, MSc[a]

KEYWORDS

- Sexual offending • Treatment • Cognitive/behavioral
- Effectiveness

While there were quite early reported attempts (even in the late nineteenth century) to modify the interests and behavior of people with sexually deviant tendencies,[1] most of these interventions were either quite limited in their scope or based on theoretical orientations that differed from most current approaches. Strictly behavioral approaches, popular in the 1960s and early 1970s[2–5] assumed that deviant dispositions were the result of simple conditioning processes.[6] It was thought, therefore, that procedures derived from animal learning studies would be sufficient to reduce these tendencies by both suppressing deviant interests[7] and enhancing appropriate sexual desires.[8] It soon became apparent that a more comprehensive approach was necessary.[9]

In North America, and in most other English-speaking countries, the currently accepted approach to the treatment of sexual offenders is some form of cognitive-behavioral therapy (CBT) with a relapse prevention (RP) component. While CBT/RP approaches have been adopted in some European countries, psychoanalysis forms the basis of treatment programs for sexual offenders in other European locations.

The specific form of CBT/RP varies considerably across programs in North America. The targeted skills, behaviors, and cognitions vary, as do the ways in which the components of treatment are presented. Some programs target a comprehensive range of issues while others have more limited goals. A review of the literature reveals that more than 50 different features of sexual offenders have been targeted in treatment across various CBT/RP programs with some programs having more, and some having fewer, RP components.

Perhaps most importantly are the quite different approaches in delivering treatment. For example, some CBT/RP clinicians advocate a strong confrontational approach to

---

[a] Rockwood Psychological Services, 403-303 Bagot Street, Kingston, Ontario, K7K 5W7, Canada
[b] Department of Psychology, Queen's University, Kingston, Ontario, K7L 3N6, Canada
* Corresponding author.
E-mail address: bill@rockwoodpsyc.com (W.L. Marshall).

Psychiatr Clin N Am 31 (2008) 681–696
doi:10.1016/j.psc.2008.06.001
0193-953X/08/$ – see front matter © 2008 Elsevier Inc. All rights reserved.

treatment delivery,[10,11] whereas others employ a more motivationally based approach that involves some degree of challenging but done in a caring and respectful way.[12,13] Some North American programs require the therapist to follow a highly detailed treatment manual while other programs have at most a "guide" for treatment providers. A psychoeducational approach, where the treatment facilitator presents the issues in a didactic format and encourages limited discussion among the clients, is adopted by some programs,[14] whereas other programs are far more psychotherapeutic in their approach.[15] Common to almost all CBT/RP programs, however, is group treatment with little in the way of individual "one-on-one" treatment.

We have attempted to overcome the problems associated with some of these approaches in devising our treatment program. We now turn to a description of our program.

THE ROCKWOOD APPROACH

The first report of our program (now called "The Rockwood Program") appeared in 1971.[16] It derived from the nascent behavior therapy approach although it also included training in relationship skills and more general social skills. Subsequently, a series of reports[13,15,17–22] illustrated the evolution of our program over the past 36 years. We have implemented this program in several Canadian federal prisons, in an outpatient community setting, and in a secure facility for mentally disordered offenders.

The evolution of the Rockwood Program continues based on available research and our clinical experience. We now address the following topics: difficulty accepting responsibility, a lack of empathy, deficient coping skills, low self-esteem, distorted beliefs and perceptions, inadequate intimacy, emotional loneliness, poor attachment styles, various general social deficits, deviant sexual interests, and how to attain a fuller, more satisfying life.[15] Many of the changes in our program, particularly over the past 15 years, have been in response to our sense that most current CBT/RP programs have at least six sets of problems: (1) a "one size fits all" approach; (2) a primarily cognitive approach; (3) a disregard of the role of therapeutic processes; (4) an exclusive focus on past history, particularly past offense history, and on developing a set of avoidance strategies for each client; (5) a failure to build the skills, attitudes, and self-regard necessary to develop a better life; and finally (6) an absence of concern about emotional issues. We discuss each of these issues separately before turning to a more detailed description of the Rockwood Program.

One Size Fits All

This involves the design of a program that is applied in the same way to all sexual offender clients. Typically such programs require therapists to follow a highly detailed treatment manual[23] and too often these programs are presented in a psychoeducational or didactic style.[14] There is now considerable evidence demonstrating the heterogeneity of sexual offenders on all issues that have been examined; as a result it is inappropriate to require all sexual offenders to rigidly follow the same treatment program. Furthermore, there is evidence indicating that therapists who adhere to a detailed treatment manual diminish their effectiveness by doing so.[24]

In the general offender treatment field, Andrews and his colleagues[25,26] have employed meta-analytic techniques to identify effective treatment principles. One of these is the *responsivity principle,* which requires the style and mode of service to be matched to the individual's abilities and learning styles. Essentially this is what the general psychotherapy literature identifies as the need for flexibility in applying treatment.[27] Accordingly, it is necessary to adjust the treatment targets, and the way issues are presented to clients, to the specific style of each individual, taking into account their current functioning.

Primarily Cognitive

Although most current sexual offender programs are described as "cognitive-behavioral," a careful examination of such programs in operation reveals that the therapists employ very few behavioral strategies. These programs focus almost exclusively on challenging the client's expressed beliefs, attitudes, and perceptions, and on providing clients with information about the relevant issues. We[28] have provided evidence showing that various behavioral strategies are effective components of an overall treatment approach. For example, we have clients role-play anticipated problematic situations (eg, situations requiring them to be assertive); we have them practice, in real-life situations, newly acquired skills (eg, social relationship skills) so that generalization will occur; we use shaping (ie, the encouragement of each small step toward a goal of enhanced skilled behavior); we ignore inappropriate behaviors or the expression of inappropriate thoughts; and we have the therapist model appropriate behaviors and attitudes. Surprisingly these well-established behavioral procedures are often absent from so-called cognitive-behavioral programs and yet many sexual offender clients do not have the educational background to respond to a strictly cognitive approach.

Even within the cognitive aspects of many CBT approaches, we have reservations. For example, it is almost universally accepted that treatment with sexual offenders should attempt to overcome what are referred to as aspects of denial (ie, client claims he did not commit an offense) and minimization (ie, client claims it was not his fault, or it was consenting sex, or he did no harm). Surprisingly, neither denial nor minimizations are related to the propensity to re-offend.[29,30] More importantly, many CBT therapists when challenging denial and minimization adopt a confrontational approach that is sometimes quite aggressive, and this is typically done at the very beginning of treatment. If the goal is to get offenders to take responsibility for their lives (including their past aberrant behavior), then we cannot expect to see changes until the client learns to trust the therapist. The early stages of treatment should emphasize a motivational approach.[31] Challenging clients at the onset of treatment seems certain to delay the development of trust and may even preclude its development. We have found that being supportive, and displaying warmth and empathy, without being challenging too early in treatment, frequently results in the clients expressing responsibility without much promoting from the therapist.

Therapeutic Processes

Our psychotherapeutic colleagues working with other populations have long maintained that the relationship between the client and therapist establishes the basis for mutual trust.[32–36] It is this trust that provides clients with the confidence to explore various possibilities including taking responsibility for their actions both past and future. Good-quality client-therapist relationships result from various features of the therapist's behavior.[37] Our research has shown that in treatment with sexual offenders, benefits are derived only when the therapist displays support, empathy, and warmth, and when clients are encouraged for small steps in the right direction.[38,39] Other researchers working with sexual offenders have found that group cohesion and expressiveness facilitate the attainment of treatment goals.[40,41]

Focus on Avoidance

One of the main foci in CBT/RP treatment of sexual offenders, is to explore in detail all of the client's past offending behavior to derive what is called an "offense pathway" or "offense cycle." It is assumed that a common chain of thoughts, feelings, and behaviors characterizes all the offenses of each individual client, and that it is only by making this chain explicit that the offender can develop strategies to avoid future offending. Plans to reduce the likelihood of re-offending after discharge from treatment are then identified. Unfortunately, however, the plans generated from CBT/RP programs typically focus only on situations or persons the client should avoid. Sometimes these avoidance plans are so comprehensive that the client's postrelease life is so markedly constricted that the client is unlikely to derive any sense of freedom or satisfaction from it.

There is now a substantial body of evidence indicating that avoidance goals are rarely maintained even under the best of conditions, but almost never maintained when life is experienced as unsatisfying.[42,43] Mann and colleagues[44] demonstrated, within sexual offender treatment, that only those clients who were encouraged to develop approach goals, rather than avoidance goals, were fully engaged in treatment, completed all their between-sessions practice, were willing to disclose problems, and were judged to be genuinely motivated to remain offense-free. Approach goals, in this context, refer to developing plans to build a better life involving behaviors that are exclusive of offending. These approach goals are aimed at assisting clients in fulfilling their potential for a prosocial and satisfying life.

Building Skills for a Better Life

Even as early as 1971, we[16] realized that focusing treatment on simply eliminating pro-offending attitudes and desires would be unlikely to reduce the subsequent propensity to re-offend. Since that time, we have progressively changed the focus of our treatment to include overcoming loneliness and intimacy deficits by developing a more secure attachment style; establishing a strong sense of self-worth; increasing the capacity to express empathy; improving coping skills; reducing shame; and instilling behavioral, emotional, and sexual self-regulatory skills.[15] Collectively, these changes have been aimed at moving the focus away from the client's past and the corollary development of avoidance plans, toward increasing skills, attitudes, and self-regulation so that a more fulfilling life can be achieved.

The *Good Lives Model*[45,46] rests on a vast body of research demonstrating that all people strive to achieve satisfactory functioning across several areas: healthy living, knowledge, mastery in play and work, autonomy and self-directedness, inner peace, effective relationships, involvement in community, spirituality, happiness, and creativity. In applying the *Good Lives Model* to the treatment of sexual offenders, the therapist works collaboratively with each client to develop a limited set of personalized goals consistent with individual interests and abilities.[47,48] Once these goals have been established, the client is helped to identify the steps needed to achieve the goals, including strategies for acquiring whatever skills are necessary to take these first steps. The aim is to start clients on this road to satisfaction by equipping them with the skills, knowledge, and self-confidence to continue striving toward fulfillment after discharge from treatment.[49]

Consistent with this emphasis on developing a better life, one of the main targets of our program involves assisting offenders in overcoming intimacy deficits and corresponding feelings of emotional loneliness. To do this we first explore the attachment they experienced (or did not experience) with their primary caregivers; such attachments are typically poor among our clients. Sexual offenders characteristically experience physical, sexual, and emotional abuse or neglect in their childhoods.[50,51] Once we have established the origins of our clients' poor attachments, we explore their adult experiences in relationships. This serves to detect the deficient style they bring to these relationships. On the basis of this analysis we can then train them in the skills, attitudes, and self-confidence necessary to enact a more secure attachment style.

This approach, however, is effective only if done within a secure attachment bond between the therapist and client. Such a secure relationship with the therapist provides clients with the confidence to explore the relevant issues and gives them the courage to enact new, more effective, behaviors with other people.

Emotional Issues

There is now evidence indicating that sexual offenders have serious deficits in self-regulation.[52] Effective self-regulation allows people to order their lives in such a way that they can successfully achieve the goals they seek (in the case of our program, the goals of the client's personalized good life plan). In the general psychological literature it has been shown that control over emotions is essential to the development of effective self-regulation.[53] Affective dysregulation does not permit clients to focus on their plans and on behaving in ways necessary to achieve these plans.[54] In addition, emotional lability diverts clients from considering the long-term effects of their actions and directs attention to the achievement of immediate satisfaction.[55] For sexual offenders, this attention to immediate satisfaction may result in the pursuit of sexual gratification. Consistent with these concerns about emotional dysregulation, acute emotional states have been found to predict the immediate likelihood of a sexual re-offense.[56]

Deficits in both behavioral and emotional self-regulation are implicated in all types of criminal behavior, in the inappropriate expression of sexual behavior, the abuse of alcohol or drugs, and in the unsatisfactory formation of attachment relationships.[53,57] Since emotional dysregulation crucially underpins both general and sexual self-regulation, then clearly this must be a target in treatment with sexual offenders. CBT/RP therapists have typically paid little attention to the emotional processes that occur during the treatment of sexual offenders.

There are several reasons why targeting emotional regulation is important in the treatment of sexual offenders. First, as we have noted, there is evidence that sexual offenders have deficits in self-regulation, which depends on emotional regulation. Second, sexual offenders have been shown to have problems accurately recognizing emotions in others,[58] stemming from their difficulties in identifying their own emotions. If clients cannot recognize their own emotional states, they are unlikely to be able to regulate their emotional expressions. Third, there is evidence that the expression of emotions during therapy is significantly predictive of positive gains being derived from sexual offender treatment.[40,41,59] Most importantly, Pfäfflin and colleagues[59] found that when the therapist and client maintain their interactions at a strictly cognitive level, the desired changes do not occur; it is only when cognitions and emotions occur in synchrony that treatment goals are achieved. As a consequence, we encourage and facilitate the expression of emotions in our clients.[15] While we have specific exercises to achieve this, we also prompt clients to identify their emotions during all aspects of treatment and we encourage any sign of emotional expression.

THE ROCKWOOD PROGRAM

Since much of our treatment approach has already been described in the preceding sections, we will simply outline the target problems we address and some of the specific procedures we employ to deal with each problem area.

The program operates in a group therapy format led by one therapist. Individual sessions are scheduled only when necessary to deal with problems arising in the group context that cannot be resolved within the group. Otherwise, we do no direct therapy on an individual basis. Groups meet twice each week for 3-hour sessions with a 10-minute break in the middle of each session. There are 10 offenders in each group and the groups all operate on an open-ended (or rolling) format. This allows each offender to progress at a pace that fits with the magnitude and complexity of each person's problems and that suits each person's personal style and learning capacity.

This flexibility allows us to keep clients in treatment until they achieve the goals of the program. It also means we can adjust our approach to suit clients with serious personality disorders. As a result, clients remain in our program for an average of 4 months (range, 3 to 6 months). It is important to note, however, that our clients are typically involved in other programs addressing their additional needs such as anger management, substance abuse, and antisocial thinking. Thus, their overall time in sexual offender specific treatment is 200 hours,[60] but the time in adjunct programs raises their time spent in overall treatment to 400 to 600 hours.

TARGETS OF TREATMENT
Life History

Early in treatment all clients must write a list of the main facts of their lives from childhood, through adolescence, early adulthood, mid-life, and older age (where each area is relevant). Clients are told that within each age span they are to note successes and problems: in relationships, sexual activities, education, work, leisure, and health, as well as any other issues the clients consider relevant. Problems and successes identified in the autobiography are discussed in the group, which begins the process of identifying the specific issues to be targeted over the course of treatment. Among the most frequent issues appearing in these autobiographies are problematic attachments with caregivers during childhood; sexual, physical, or emotional abuse; low self-worth; sexual difficulties or aberrations; poor coping responses to difficulties; adult relationship difficulties; a failure to take responsibility for their actions; and poor self-regulation skills. Most importantly, these autobiographies identify a range of strengths for each client, which assists the therapist in convincing clients that they have the capacity (ie, the self-efficacy) to change.

Self-Worth

First we assist clients in identifying their current level of self-esteem across various domains of functioning, and then we explore with each client the likely origins of this poor self-regard. We then implement strategies that we[61,62] have demonstrated to be effective in enhancing self-worth. We repeatedly remind our clients that they are distinct from their offending behavior and we repeatedly point to their strengths. This is aimed at overcoming the shame sexual offenders typically express when they first enter treatment.[63] Feelings of shame reflect an attribution for inappropriate behaviors to a defect in the person (ie, "I am a bad person" or "I am a pedophile"), and this prevents the person from believing that change is possible.[64] Guilt, on the other hand, reflects an attribution for bad behavior to poor decision-making (ie, "I am capable of good behavior but made a poor choice"), and this encourages a belief in the possibility of change.[64] Thus, focusing on the clients' strengths and enhancing their sense of self-worth, while treating them respectfully, should reduce shame and facilitate engagement in the change process.

Sexual offenders are encouraged throughout treatment to engage in all positive opportunities (eg, evening leisure activities, weekend groups run by volunteers, social activities, and any legitimate pleasurable opportunities) available in prison. Finally, we assist clients individually to identify positive qualities about themselves that are apparent in each of several domains of functioning (eg, as a friend, as a family member, at work, at play, and in terms of knowledge and interests). Clients record these positive qualities on pocket-sized cards that are always carried with them; clients read each quality repeatedly every day throughout treatment.

Acceptance of Responsibility

Underlying the tendency of clients to deny or minimize their personal responsibility for their choices and actions is their deep-seated lack of self-worth and the associated sense of shame. Thus, enhancing self-worth, reducing shame, and providing clients with the skills and attitudes necessary to meet their needs prosocially, all contribute to their gradual acceptance of responsibility; as does the trust engendered by the therapist who shows acceptance of them but not of their offensive behaviors.

Clients are assisted in identifying perceptions, attitudes, and beliefs, as well as the schema underlying them, that allow them to diminish their responsibility. They are encouraged to accept that all people have flaws so they do not have to be perfect to be acceptable and to function well. We point out to clients that a failure to accept responsibility results in costs to themselves as well as to others and we encourage them to generate a cost-benefit analysis of accepting versus failing to accept responsibility for their actions. Any small steps in the direction of taking responsibility are rewarded with encouragement, compliments, and appropriate body language by the therapist.

Offense Pathways

Part of the process involved in accepting responsibility includes the client providing a description of the events preceding the offense. Here, unlike most CBT/RP therapists, we are not particularly interested in the details of the offense but rather in the factors that led each client to offend. We speak of these as "background factors" and they often include persistent low self-worth, problems in relationships, anger (usually at women), perceived failures, acute mood states, and intoxication. These issues have been identified as "dynamic risk factors" for sexual offenders,[56] and the presence of these problems has been shown to prompt deviant fantasizing among incarcerated sexual offenders.[65–67] Clients are made aware that these background factors make them vulnerable to taking more precise steps toward offending. These steps typically involve rationalizing or justifying an attempt to offend, generating deviant sexual thoughts, seeking out a victim, and setting the occasion for offending by arranging to be alone with a potential victim.[68]

Once we have identified the personally relevant background factors, we can discuss these issues with the clients to design strategies and teach behaviors that will allow the client to take an action other than offending. The remaining parts of the program, up to release planning, address these identified background factors by providing the required training in skills and in modifying dysfunctional attitudes, beliefs, and schema.

Coping Skills

Sexual offenders have been shown to have poor coping styles[69–71] and deficiencies in their capacity to deal with specific problem situations.[72] A failure to deal effectively with stressors or other problematic issues leads people to engage in unacceptable behaviors or to experience distress.[73,74] It is necessary, therefore, to train sexual offenders in more effective coping skills and strategies.

As a first step, we describe what is known about coping styles, their function, and the skills that underlie effective coping. Discussions focus on each client's past responses to problems that generated distress. These responses are then analyzed to reveal to clients how their responses affected them in a negative way and led to offending behavior. Possible alternative responses are identified and clients role-play these alternatives along with their original responses. Clients are then assisted in weighing the likely value of each response both in terms of potential behavioral outcomes and the emotional consequences to themselves. Reverse role-plays are enacted to allow clients to see how other people might perceive their responses.

Practice and discussions assist each client in recognizing the emotional ups-and-downs that poor coping causes. When disruptive emotional responses to the mismanagement of stress (such as anger, anxiety, and dysphoric mood) are identified as typical consequences, clients are helped, within role-plays and discussion, to recognize the dysfunctional nature of their cognitive and behavioral responses. Allowing clients to vent their feelings, within reasonable limits, helps them experience their emotions without negative consequences and this contributes to developing better emotional regulation, which, in turn, increases overall self-regulatory skills. We[72] have demonstrated that this approach results in enhanced capacities to cope with problems.

Relationship Issues

We[75,76] have argued that sexual offenders turn to aberrant ways to meet their perceived needs because they lack the skills, attitudes, and self-confidence necessary to function effectively in adult relationships. In our view, these problems are so central to sexual offending that targeting them is a centerpiece in our treatment program.

Since we have elsewhere detailed our approach to these issues,[15,18,77] we will simply mention here the specific targets of this component. The topics addressed within this segment include the need for mutual respect and equality in relationships, the nature and value of empathy, communication skills, issues surrounding attachment and intimacy, the importance of carefully selecting a partner, the factors involved in maintaining relationships, and the impact of jealousy on effective relationships. We[77] have demonstrated that this approach effectively enhances the intimacy skills of sexual offenders and reduces their feelings of emotional loneliness.

Sexual Interests

As noted earlier, early behavioral approaches to the treatment of sexual offenders focused almost exclusively on the modification of sexual interests. While the emphasis on this issue has been significantly reduced, it still holds a place in most programs.[78] A significant number of sexual offenders do display deviant arousal patterns at phallometric assessments,[79] although far from all of them. For those who do display deviance there may be a need to implement procedures to modify these interests. The recent influx of child pornography users also raises the possibility that additional resources directed at modifying deviant interests may be needed. Two aspects of our program are expected to effectively address these issues: (1) our overall program has several elements (eg, enhancement of self-esteem, reduction of shame, improved coping skills, better relationship skills, training in effective sexual functioning, and increased empathy) that can be expected to influence sexual interests; and (2) a combination of behavioral procedures and pharmacologic interventions are implemented when the overall program does not produce changes in such interests.

Within the context of focusing on sexual interests (deviant and appropriate), we first discuss the broad range of human sexual behavior, particularly those behaviors that facilitate the sexual satisfaction of both members of a consenting adult relationship.[80,81] Rather than focusing only on eliminating deviant sexual interests, our broader approach also concentrates on enhancing normative sexual functioning.

The underlying belief that guides this is that sexual offenders pursue deviant acts because normative sexual behaviors do not produce for them the level of satisfaction that they (and all others) seek. This failure to achieve satisfaction within an appropriate sexual relationship is due, we believe to the client's lack of the skills, attitudes and beliefs, knowledge, and self-confidence necessary to produce a satisfying relationship. If our clients acquire a satisfactory level of competence across these areas, their deviant interests should be sufficiently attenuated. We have demonstrated that this actually happens. Marshall[82] selected a highly deviant group of child molesters based on their offense history (eg, all of them had numerous victims, were sexually very intrusive with their victims, and used strongly coercive tactics to gain victim compliance). From among these deviant offenders, Marshall then selected only those who also displayed strong deviant sexual arousal at phallometric evaluation. For the clients in this particular study, treatment did not directly address deviant sexual interests, but covered all other issues outlined in this issue. At posttreatment phallometric assessments their sexual interests had been normalized, and none of them have re-offended after 10 years at risk in the community.

Our main goals in this segment of treatment, then, are not usually to directly modify deviant sexual interests but rather to create greater comfort with sexuality, reduce prudishness, delineate appropriate sexual boundaries, and increase general sexual knowledge. In particular, our aim is to enhance the skills, behaviors, and attitudes that facilitate sexual satisfaction, which in turn relates to relationship satisfaction and life satisfaction.[83] We point out to clients that all the issues discussed in the human sexuality component are relevant to the issues raised in the treatment segment dealing with intimacy, attachment style, and relationships. The therapist helps clients to integrate these two sets of issues.

There are, however, some sexual offenders who are so deviant, they require more direct intervention. Sexual sadists, for example, have deeply entrenched deviant sexual scripts that are typically resistant to our other interventions.[84,85] For these and other clients who have a deeply entrenched deviant fantasy life, we employ two approaches. These two approaches, it is important to note, are done in such a way that clients view them as an embedded part of the overall program.

First, we teach the client ways to self-modify deviant thoughts during masturbation.[86] If these masturbatory reconditioning strategies are insufficiently effective, then we place the client on an antiandrogen; as a condition of parole, the client may be required to remain on the medication after release. In addition we[87,88] have shown that some 30% to 40% of sexual offenders meet criteria for what has been variously called "sexual addiction," "sexual compulsivity," or "hypersexuality." For these clients, one of the selective serotonin reuptake inhibitors is employed as an adjunct to the psychological treatment.

Self-Management Plans

The final segment of our treatment integrates what has already been covered and assists each client in identifying a limited list of potential risks to be avoided in the future, and in specifying goals for a future better life. They also develop plans to achieve these latter goals and generate a realistic set of release plans.

We limit the risks to be avoided to usually only one or two crucial potential problems. For example, a child molester should never allow himself to be alone with a child, a rapist should avoid placing himself in a situation where he has ready access to a victim, an offender whose crimes were committed while intoxicated should aim for abstinence from the problem drug. Too many programs focus on risk avoidance by severely restricting released offenders, so that the clients cannot build a meaningful life. These excessive restrictions, ironically, place sexual offenders at greater risk to re-offend. In addition to simply identifying one or two avoidance strategies to minimize risk, we alert clients to the steps they should take if one of their relevant background factors emerges. For example, if an acute mood was part of the background that precipitated previous offenses, then the client needs to develop strategies for dealing with acute problematic moods occurring after discharge from treatment. Our goal here is to get clients to look beyond what has put them at risk in the past and to develop a generic disposition toward future possible risks. This disposition would allow them to recognize novel risk situations so that they could avoid, or escape from, these situations should they occur.

Our main focus in this final segment of treatment, however, is on helping each client develop self-relevant *Good Life* plans.[45,89] It has been shown that the attainment of the goods identified in research on the good life depends on internal conditions (skills and capacities) and external conditions (opportunities and support). When the goals of a good life are not met, at least to a reasonable degree, the person will have a poorly integrated sense of self, will experience frustration, feel unsatisfied, helpless, and hopeless, and is likely to seek satisfaction in maladaptive ways.[48]

Research on the *Good Lives Model*[45,46,90,91] has generated nine domains of functioning wherein individuals strive for fulfillment across several areas of functioning (see earlier section). The descriptor "good lives" is used because there is no one "good life" that all people should adopt. Rather, individual interests, abilities, and opportunities define each person's own "good life." Thus, for each individual a unique set of good life plans should be articulated. No individuals are expected to fulfill their potential in all these domains; indeed, from this view, life is seen as a process of continually striving toward fulfillment in each domain.

One of the important implications for treatment providers of this notion of a life-long striving toward fulfillment, is that it is our responsibility to bring our clients far enough along the road to achieving the skills, attitudes, and plans necessary for them to continue to develop on their own and self-manage their lives after discharge. Our clients need not function at optimal levels on the treatment goals before release; we aim at a level of overall functioning that is close enough to normative to allow them to continue to build their strengths upon return to the community. Too many treatment programs require high levels of functioning before they are willing to discharge sexual offenders and, as a result, they keep clients in treatment too long. This is unwise, as there are reasons to believe that overtreating sexual offenders may actually increase rather than decrease their level of risk.

In this aspect of treatment, the therapist helps each client develop his own individualized good life plan. As a creative goal, a reasonably high functioning client might identify wanting to become a portrait photographer. With the group's help, facilitated by the therapist, he identifies the skills he will need, where and how he might acquire these skills, and how much money he will need to buy equipment and enroll in a course. He then considers how he can generate the necessary funds and how he can fit learning the skills into his need to fulfill his other responsibilities. For a lower functioning client, the creativity goal differs. One of our clients, for example, had always wanted to build model airplanes. This seemed to be well within his skills, so we worked with him to define the ways he could achieve this goal.

As we have seen, domains of functioning other than creativity need to be explored with each client, but it is best not to overwhelm clients with too many specific goals. We typically work only on three or four domains with each client. Characteristically we target domains such as work, leisure (including creativity), and relationships. We also describe the other areas so they can pursue them in the future if they wish.

Fitting in with the good lives plans, each client identifies two groups of people who can support his continued pursuit of his good life upon his discharge. These groups can also help the client avoid risks. A group of professionals, such as treatment providers, a parole/probation officer, or a clergyman, are identified and their roles are clarified. Similarly, friends, family, or workmates can serve as a nonprofessional group with their specific contributions being described. Typically the latter group can help the client to continue to work on developing good life plans. It has been shown that for sexual offenders, good supports can contribute to an offense-free life.[56]

Finally, each client develops release plans concerning what sort of job he will seek, where he will live and, importantly, how he intends to fill his leisure time. Inactivity or boredom can be important risk factors for sexual offenders so being occupied at a reasonable job and in enjoyable leisure activities is quite important. Of course the client is guided to choose jobs, residence, and leisure pursuits that do not expose him to risks to re-offend.

TREATMENT EFFECTS

Hanson and colleagues[92] and Lösel and Schmucker[93] have reported meta-analyses of as many as 69 outcome studies of sexual offender treatment involving thousands of offenders. Both reports found significant beneficial effects for sexual offender treatment but only for those programs that followed current CBT practices. Overall, the effect sizes (ES) produced by CBT programs were reasonable (ES = 0.28) but could certainly be better.

We[94] recently evaluated the program we have operated in a Canadian prison setting for the past 15 years. In our evaluation, 534 treated sexual offenders had been released into the community for an average of 5.4 years (48% had been in the community for over 6 years). Only 3.2% had sexually re-offended, whereas the expected rate (based on an estimate derived from the offenders' actuarial risk levels) was 16.8%. This produces an ES of 1.0, which is four times greater than the ES reported in the meta-analyses of Hanson and colleagues[92] and Lösel and Schmucker.[93]

The majority of programs entering the meta-analyses of Hanson and colleagues and Lösel and Schmucker were typical CBT/RP programs that were quite structured, delivered in the same way to all clients, primarily focused on past deviance and future avoidance plans, and with little concern for therapeutic processes. Our program with its adaptation to each client, a focus on the future and on developing a more fulfilling life, and an emphasis on the importance of the therapeutic processes, is quite different from other CBT/RP programs. On this point it is relevant to note that none of the clients in our program who scored in the psychopathic range on Hare's[95] Psychopathy Checklist-Revised, or who suffered from any other personality disorder, were found to have re-offended. No other program reported in the literature has been successful in treating psychopaths, and most programs consider clients with other personality problems to be difficult to treat.

These observations, we believe, attest to the value of our program's ability to adjust to the idiosyncratic features of our clients (ie, in meeting the "responsivity" principle) and focusing treatment on the individually determined issues of each client. The evidence from our outcome study, then, suggests that our positive and flexible approach may be more effective than traditional CBT/RP programs.

REFERENCES

1. Laws DR, Marshall WL. A brief history of behavioral and cognitive-behavioral approaches to sexual offender treatment: Part 1. Early developments. Sex Abuse 2003;15:75–92.
2. Abel GG, Levis D, Clancy J. Aversion therapy applied to taped sequences of deviant behavior in exhibitionism and other sexual deviations: a preliminary report. J Behav Ther Exp Psychiatry 1970;1:58–66.
3. Bancroft JHJ, Marks I. Electric aversion therapy of sexual deviations. Proc R Soc Med 1968;61:796–9.
4. Marks IM, Gelder JG, Bancroft JHJ. Sexual deviants two years after electric aversion therapy. Br J Psychiatry 1970;117:173–85.
5. Serber M. Shame aversion therapy. J Behav Ther Exp Psychiatry 1970;1:213–5.
6. McGuire RJ, Carlisle JM, Young BG. Sexual deviations as conditioned behaviour: a hypothesis. Behav Res Ther 1965;3:185–90.
7. Bond IK, Evans DR. Avoidance therapy: its use in two cases of underwear fetishism. CMAJ (Ottawa) 1967;96:1160–2.
8. Marquis JM. Orgasmic reconditioning: changing sexual object choice through controlling masturbation fantasies. J Behav Ther Exp Psychiatry 1970;1:263–71.
9. Marshall WL, Laws DR. A brief history of behavioral and cognitive behavioral approaches to sexual offender treatment: Part 2. The modern era. Sex Abuse 2003; 15:93–120.
10. Salter AG. Treating child sex offenders and victims: a practical guide. Thousand Oaks (CA): Sage Publications; 1988.
11. Wyre R. Working with the paedophile. In: Farrell M, editor. Understanding the paedophile. London: ISTD/The Portman Clinic; 1989. p. 17–23.
12. Mann RE, Ginsberg JID, Weekes JR. Motivational interviewing with offenders. In: McMurran M, editor. Motivating offenders to change: a guide to enhancing engagement in therapy. Chichester (UK): John Wiley & Sons; 2002. p. 87–102.
13. Marshall WL, Ward T, Mann RE, et al. Working positively with sexual offenders: maximizing the effectiveness of treatment. J Interpers Violence 2005;20:1–19.
14. Green R. Psycho-educational modules. In: Schwartz BK, Cellini HR, editors. The sex offender: corrections, treatment and legal practice. Kingston (NJ): Civic Research Institute; 1995. p. 13.1–13.10.
15. Marshall WL, Marshall LE, Serran GA, et al. Treating sexual offenders: an integrated approach. New York: Routledge; 2006.
16. Marshall WL. A combined treatment method for certain sexual deviations. Behav Res Ther 1971;9:292–4.
17. Marshall WL. The treatment of sex offenders in a community clinic. In: Ross RR, Antonowicz DH, Dhaliwal GK, editors. Going straight: effective delinquency prevention and offender rehabilitation. Ottawa (ON): Air Training & Publications; 1995. p. 277–305.
18. Marshall WL, Anderson D, Fernandez YM. Cognitive behavioural treatment of sexual offenders. Chichester (UK): John Wiley & Sons; 1999.
19. Marshall WL, Barbaree HE. The long-term evaluation of a behavioral treatment program for child molesters. Behav Res Ther 1988;26:499–511.
20. Marshall WL, Earls CM, Segal ZV, et al. A behavioral program for the assessment and treatment of sexual aggressors. In: Craig K, McMahon R, editors. Advances in clinical behavior therapy. New York: Brunner/Mazel; 1983. p. 148–74.
21. Marshall WL, McKnight RD. An integrated treatment program for sexual offenders. Can J Psychiatry 1975;20:133–8.

22. Marshall WL, Redondo S. Control y tratamiento de la aggression sexual. In: Redondo S, editor. Delincuencio sexual y sociedad. Valencia (Spain): Ariel Publishing; 2002. p. 301–28.

23. Marques JK. An innovative treatment program for sex offenders: report to the legislature. Sacramento (CA): California Department of Mental Health; 1984.

24. Goldfried MR, Wolfe B. Psychotherapy practice and research: repairing a strained alliance. Am Psychol 1996;51:1007–16.

25. Andrews DA, Bonta J. The psychology of criminal conduct. 3rd edition. Cincinnati (OH): Anderson; 2001.

26. Gendreau P, Andrews DA. Tertiary prevention: what the meta-analyses of the offender treatment literature tell us about "what works." Canadian Journal of Criminology 1990;32:173–84.

27. Martin DJ, Garske JP, Davis MK. Relation of the therapeutic alliance with outcome and other variables: a meta-analytic review. J Consult Clin Psychol 2000;68: 438–50.

28. Fernandez YM, Shingler J, Marshall WL, et al. Putting "behavior" back into the cognitive-behavioral treatment of sexual offenders. In: Marshall WL, Fernandez YM, Marshall LE, et al, editors. Sexual offender treatment: controversial issues. Chichester (UK): John Wiley & Sons; 2006. p. 211–24.

29. Hanson RK, Bussière MT. Predicting relapse: a meta-analysis of sexual offender recidivism studies. J Consult Clin Psychol 1998;66:348–62.

30. Hanson RK, Morton-Bourgon K. Predictors of sexual recidivism: an updated meta-analysis. (Cat. NO. P53-1/2004-2E-PDF). Ottawa (ON): Public Works and Government Services of Canada; 2004.

31. Miller WR, Rollnick S, editors. Motivational interviewing: preparing people to change addictive behavior. 2nd edition. 3rd. New York: Guilford Press; 2002.

32. Frank JD. Therapeutic factors in psychotherapy. Am J Psychother 1971;25: 350–61.

33. Lambert MJ. The individual therapist's contribution to psychotherapy process and outcome. Clin Psychol Rev 1989;9:469–85.

34. Rogers CR. The necessary and sufficient conditions of therapeutic personality change. J Consult Psychol 1957;21:95–103.

35. Strupp HH, Hadley SW. Specific vs. nonspecific factors in psychotherapy. Arch Gen Psychiatry 1979;36:1125–36.

36. Yalom ID. The theory and practice of group psychotherapy. 3rd edition. New York: Basic Books; 1985.

37. Marshall WL, Fernandez YM, Serran GA, et al. Process variables in the treatment of sexual offenders: a review of the relevant literature. Aggression and Violent Behavior: A Review Journal 2003;8:205–34.

38. Marshall WL, Serran GA, Fernandez YM, et al. Therapist characteristics in the treatment of sexual offenders: tentative data on their relationship with indices of behaviour change. Journal of Sexual Aggression 2003;9:25–30.

39. Marshall WL, Serran GA, Moulden J, et al. Therapist features in sexual offender treatment: their reliable identification and influence on behaviour change. Clin Psychol Psychother 2002;9:395–405.

40. Beech AR, Fordham AS. Therapeutic climate of sexual offender treatment programs. Sex Abuse 1997;9:219–37.

41. Beech AR, Hamilton-Giachritsis CE. Relationship between therapeutic climate and treatment outcome in group-based sexual offender treatment programs. Sex Abuse 2005;17:127–40.

42. Emmons RA. Striving and feeling: personal goals and subjective well-being. In: Gollwitzer PM, Bargh JA, editors. The psychology of action: linking cognition and motivation to behavior. New York: Guilford Press; 1996. p. 313–37.

43. Gollwitzer PM, Bargh JA, editors. The psychology of action: linking cognition and motivation to behavior. New York: Guilford Press; 1996.

44. Mann RE, Webster SD, Scholfield C, et al. Approach versus avoidance goals in relapse prevention with sexual offenders. Sex Abuse 2004;16:65–75.

45. Deci WL, Ryan RM. The "what" and "why" of goal pursuits: human needs and the self-determination of behavior. Psychol Inq 2000;1:227–68.

46. Emmons RA. The psychology of ultimate concerns. New York: Guilford Press; 1999.

47. Ward T. Good lives and the rehabilitation of offenders: promises and problems. Aggression and Violent Behavior: A Review Journal 2002;7:513–28.

48. Ward T, Stewart CA. Good lives and the rehabilitation of sexual offenders. In: Ward T, Laws DR, Hudson SM, editors. Sexual deviance: issues and controversies. Thousands Oaks (CA): Sage Publications; 2003. p. 22–44.

49. Ward T, Marshall WL. Good lives, aetiology and the rehabilitation of sex offenders: a bridging theory. Journal of Sexual Aggression 2004;10:153–69.

50. Marshall WL, Marshall LE. The origins of sexual offending. Trauma, Violence, Abuse: A Review Journal 2000;1:250–63.

51. Starzyk KB, Marshall WL. Childhood, family, and personological risk factors for sexual offending. Aggression and Violent Behavior: A Review Journal 2003;8: 93–105.

52. Ward T, Hudson SM. A self-regulation model of relapse prevention. In: Laws DR, Hudson SM, Ward T, editors. Remaking relapse prevention with sex offenders: a sourcebook. Thousand Oaks (CA): Sage Publications; 2000. p. 79–101.

53. Baumeister RF, Vohs KD, editors. Handbook of self-regulation: research, theory, and applications. New York: Guilford Press; 2004.

54. Rimé B. Interpersonal emotion regulation. In: Gross JJ, editor. Handbook of emotion regulation. New York: Guilford Press; 2007. p. 466–85.

55. Rothbart MK, Sheese BE. Temperament and emotion regulation. In: Gross JJ, editor. Handbook of emotion regulation. New York: Guilford Press; 2007. p. 331–50.

56. Hanson RK, Harris AJR. Where should we intervene? Dynamic predictors of sex offender recidivism. Crim Justice Behav 2000;27:6–35.

57. Gross JJ, editor. Handbook of emotion regulation. New York: Guilford Press; 2007.

58. Hudson SM, Marshall WL, Wales DS, et al. Emotional recognition skills of sex offenders. Annals of Sex Research 1993;6:199–211.

59. Pfäfflin F, Böhmer M, Cornehl S, et al. What happens in therapy with sexual offenders? A model of process research. Sex Abuse 2005;17:141–51.

60. Marshall WL, Yates PM. Comment on Mailloux, et al.'s (2003) study: "Dosage of treatment of sexual offenders: Are we overprescribing?". International Journal of Offender Treatment and Comparative Criminology 2005;49:221–4.

61. Marshall WL, Champagne F, Sturgeon C, et al. Increasing the self-esteem of child molesters. Sex Abuse 1997;9:321–33.

62. Marshall WL, Christie MM. The enhancement of social self-esteem. Canadian Counsellor 1982;16:82–9.

63. Marshall WL, Marshall LE. Shame, self-esteem, and empathy: their relevance for sexual offender treatment. Psychology, Crime & Law, in press.

64. Tangney JP, Dearing RL. Shame and guilt. New York: Guilford Press; 2002.

65. Looman J. Mood, conflict, and deviant sexual fantasies. In: Schwartz BK, editor, The sex offender: theoretical advances, treating special populations and legal developments, vol. III. Kingston (NJ): Civic Research Institute; 1999. p. 3.1–3.11.

66. McKibben A, Proulx J, Lusignan R. Relationships between conflict, affect and deviant sexual behaviors in rapists and pedophiles. Behav Res Ther 1994;32:571–5.

67. Proulx J, McKibben A, Lusignan R. Relationships between affective components and sexual behaviors in sexual aggressors. Sex Abuse 1996;8:279–89.

68. Ward T, Louden K, Hudson SM, et al. A descriptive model of the offense chain for child molesters. Journal of Interpersonal Violence 1995;10:452–72.

69. Cortoni FA, Marshall WL. Sex as a coping strategy and its relationship to juvenile sexual history and intimacy in sexual offenders. Sex Abuse 2001;13:27–43.

70. Marshall WL, Serran GA, Cortoni FA. Childhood attachments, sexual abuse, and their relationship to adult coping in child molesters. Sex Abuse 2000;12:17–26.

71. Neidigh LW, Tomiko R. The coping strategies of child sexual abusers. J Sex Educ Ther 1991;17:103–10.

72. Serran GA, Firestone P, Marshall WL, et al. Changes in coping following treatment for child molesters. Journal of Interpersonal Violence 2007;22:1199–210.

73. Lazarus RS. Toward better research on stress and coping. Am Psychol 2000;55: 665–73.

74. Zeinder M, Endler NS. Handbook of coping: theory, research, applications. New York: John Wiley & Sons; 1996.

75. Marshall WL. Intimacy, loneliness, and sexual offenders. Behav Res Ther 1989; 27:491–503.

76. Marshall WL. The role of attachment, intimacy, and loneliness in the etiology and maintenance of sexual offending. Sex Marital Ther 1993;8:109–21.

77. Marshall WL, Bryce P, Hudson SM, et al. The enhancement of intimacy and the reduction of loneliness among child molesters. J Fam Violence 1996;11:219–35.

78. McGrath RJ, Cumming GF, Burchard BL. Current practices and trends in sexual abuser management: safer society 2002 nationwide survey. Brandon (VT): Safer Society Press; 2003.

79. Marshall WL, Fernandez YM. Phallometric testing with sexual offenders: theory, research, and practice. Brandon (VT): Safer Society Press; 2003.

80. Hyde JS, DeLamater JD, Byers ES, editors. Understanding human sexuality. 2nd edition. Toronto: McGraw-Hill Ryerson; 2004.

81. Regan PC. Love relationships. In: Szuchman LT, Muscarella F, editors. Psychological perspectives on human sexuality. New York: John Wiley & Sons; 2000. p. 232–82.

82. Marshall WL. The relationship between self-esteem and deviant sexual arousal in nonfamilial child molesters. Behav Modif 1997;12:86–96.

83. Rathus SA, Nevid JS, Fichner-Rathus L, editors. Human sexuality in a world of diversity. 4th edition. Boston: Allyn and Bacon; 2000.

84. Marshall WL, Hucker SJ. Sexual sadism: its features and treatment. In: McNulty RD, editor. Sex and sexuality, Sexual deviation and sexual offenses, vol. 3. Westport (CT): Greenwood Publishing; 2006. p. 227–50.

85. Proulx J, Blais E, Beauregard É, et al. Sadistic sexual offenders. In: Proulx J, Beauregard É, Cusson M, editors. Sexual murderers: a comparative analysis and new perspective. Chichester (UK): John Wiley & Sons; 2007. p. 107–22.

86. Marshall WL, O'Brien MD, Marshall LE. Modifying sexual interests. In: AR Beech, LA Craig, KD Browne, editors. Assessment and treatment of sex offenders: a handbook. John Wiley & Sons, in press.

87. Marshall LE, O'Brien MD, Marshall WL. Sexual addiction in incarcerated sexual offenders. In: AR Beech, LA Craig, KD Browne, editors. Assessment and treatment of sex offenders: a handbook. Chichester (UK): John Wiley & Sons, in press.

88. O'Brien MD, Marshall LE, Marshall WL. Sexual addiction. In: DL Rowland, L Incrocci, editors. Handbook of sexual and gender identity disorders. New York: John Wiley & Sons, in press.

89. Schmuck P, Sheldon KM, editors. Life goals and well-being. Toronto: Hogrefe & Huber; 2001.

90. Austin JT, Vancouver JB. Goal constructs in psychology: structure, process, and content. Psychol Bull 1996;120:338–75.

91. Rasmussen DB. Human flourishing and the appeal to human nature. In: Paul EF, Miller FD, Paul J, editors. Human flourishing. New York: Cambridge University; 1999. p. 1–43.

92. Hanson RK, Gordon A, Harris AJR, et al. First report of the collaborative outcome data project on the effectiveness of psychological treatment of sexual offenders. Sex Abuse 2002;14:169–95.

93. Lösel F, Schmucker M. The effectiveness of treatment for sexual offenders: a comprehensive meta-analysis. Journal of Experimental Criminology 2005;1:1–29.

94. Marshall LE, Marshall WL. Outcome data from Bath Institution's Sexual Offender Treatment Program. Paper in preparation.

95. Hare RD. Manual for the Hare psychopathy checklist-revised. Toronto: Multi-Health Systems; 1991.

Treatment of Compulsive Cybersex Behavior

Stephen Southern, EdD

KEYWORDS

- Compulsive cybersex • Pornography • Sexual abuse
- Sexual addiction • Sexual compulsivity

Ongoing expansion of the Internet and proliferation of sexually oriented sites have contributed to conditions that favor the pathogenesis of compulsive cybersex behavior. The term *cybersex* includes an array of online sexual activity associated with Internet usage: viewing erotic or pornographic images from news services, bulletin boards or Web sites; exposing explicit details of one's sex life by uploading or forwarding images or text descriptions of oneself or one's partner; interacting with sex workers employed by particular Web sites; interacting with anonymous partners through chat rooms, blogs, or other mediated contacts; meeting potential sexual partners for offline contacts; and violating interpersonal boundaries by engaging in unwanted sexually oriented contacts through e-mail, social networking sites, or other Internet venues.

In the most common, restrictive use of the term, *cybersex* refers to a sequence of visual or textual exchanges with a partner for the purposes of sexual pleasure, which frequently culminates in masturbation.[1–3] Such *cybering* behavior typically occurs between consenting partners in private spaces accessed through e-mail, instant messaging, real-time exchanges via Web sites, or other consensual means. However, cyber-contacts for purposes of sexual outlet may cause conflict or consequences to the extent they are secretive or illicit (eg, extramarital affairs) or illegal (eg, engaging minors in sexual interactions). The array of particular cybersex behaviors ranges from solitary acts through consensual interactions to coercive contacts. Problematic cybersex behavior represents a disturbance of sexual functions ordinarily associated with eroticism in intimate couples. Compulsive cybersex may be distinguished from problematic behavior based on perceptions of lack of control or choice and experiences of negative consequences by patients for whom the cybersex behavior is dystonic or unacceptable. Negative consequences of compulsive cybersex affect familial, social, and vocational functioning, as well as physical and spiritual domains.

Department of Psychology, Mississippi College, 112 Lowrey Hall, P.O. Box 4013, Clinton, MS 39058, USA
E-mail address: southern@mc.edu

Psychiatr Clin N Am 31 (2008) 697–712
doi:10.1016/j.psc.2008.06.003
0193-953X/08/$ – see front matter © 2008 Elsevier Inc. All rights reserved.

psych.theclinics.com

The potential for problems with compulsive cybersex in American society is sobering. More than half of Americans (172 million persons) regularly use the Internet with as many as a third going online for sexual purposes.[4] The cybersexual revolution contributed to the exponential growth of the World Wide Web and Internet technology. Many innovations, such as video streaming, were developed by the online sex industry.[5] An estimated 60% of all visits and commerce on the Internet were associated with sexual activities.[6] Internet sex was the third largest economic sector on the Web (following software and computers), generating $1 billion of revenue each year.[5] There is a symbiotic relationship between the rapidly growing Internet and the ongoing cybersex revolution.

According to these statistics, cybersex on the Internet is a normative experience for millions of Americans. Problems with compulsive cybersex tend to develop in vulnerable or at-risk users who are predisposed to developing obsessive preoccupation, frequent and harmful outlet, and continued online sexual behavior despite negative consequences.[5,6] Problematic cybersex has been associated with heavy Internet use defined as 20 or more hours online per week.[7]

Heavy Internet usage has been linked to a wide range of problems in clinical and nonclinical samples.[7–11] While international researchers in sexuality and new media technologies perceived educational, play, and entertainment benefits from involvement in cybersex,[12–14] other commentators emphasized the potential for harm to couples and families[15] and disinhibition of hypersexual and sex offender behavior.[16] Cooper and colleagues[7,17] have maintained a balanced view regarding potentially helpful and harmful aspects of Internet sexuality. The potential dangers of cybersex may be in the eyes of the beholder in that postmodern researchers and theorists tend to emphasize the social construction of danger, risk, and safety.[18] Nevertheless, a growing body of literature and expert opinion have implicated the potential risk of heavy Internet usage in the development of sexual and relational problems.

A study of 1504 practitioners who reported at least one client with an Internet-related problem produced an inventory of 11 types of problematic Internet experiences encountered in clinical practice.[9] Internet problems that were the primary focus of treatment are listed here in descending percentage of young and adult patients: sexual exploitation (48%), infidelity (47%), pornography (44%), overuse (40%), failed relationships (37%), fraud and deception (37%), gaming and role-playing (29%), harassment (28%), risky behavior, not otherwise specified (NOS) (28%), harmful influence (23%), and isolative-avoidant use (23%). The list of clinical problems emphasized sexual and relational issues, deception and criminal conduct, and harmful social impacts.

Cooper[19] observed that the sexual revolution of the Internet was fueled by the "Triple A Engine" of accessibility, affordability, and anonymity. Schwartz and Southern[20] described compulsive cybersex as the "new tea room" in which cruising can lead to easy anonymous and impersonal sex. The mood altering and interactive characteristics of Internet sex also predispose vulnerable users to develop problems with cybersex.[21] Cybersex may also function as dissociative reenactment by which fantasy transmutes life tragedy into triumph.[20,22]

The sights and sounds of the Internet contribute to the development of sexual fantasies that would likely not be explored through conventional means by consumers unfamiliar with pornography or sex industry participation, including women.[23,24] Women may constitute 40% of those who experience severe problems with Internet sex.[5] An early clinical study of patients seeking treatment for compulsive cybersex identified equal numbers of men and women.[21]

Other populations affected by the cybersex revolution that typically had been insulated from pornography and other sexual stimuli include juveniles at home and in the community and employees in their work settings. Since 90% of youth between 12 and 18 years old have access to the Internet,[25] they may be considered a population at risk for harmful effects associated with cybersex. The Youth Internet Safety Survey, a nationally representative sample of 1501 10- to 17-year-olds who used the Internet regularly, established that within a year, 19% reported an unwanted sexual solicitation, 25% reported unwanted exposure to sexual material, and 6% had been harassed online.[26] Data from the national survey revealed that many youth sought pornography (online and offline) with most being male (95%) and 14 years of age or older (87%).[25,26] On the positive side, recent research that tracked trends in youth reports of Internet sexual activity between 2000 and 2005 found that sexual solicitations of boys and girls in all age groups had declined.[27] The authors concluded that education programs and law enforcement efforts were reducing predatory contacts for all groups except low-income, minority youth.[27] There were also troubling increases in unwanted exposure to pornography, attributed to aggressive marketing strategies by pornography vendors.[27]

Children and adolescents experience direct and indirect effects of exposure to Internet pornography, which brings explicit materials into homes, schools, and community settings.[28,29] Indirect exposure to the compulsive cybersex activity of family members and significant others can produce negative impacts such as shame, fear, or loss, as well as family upheaval.[29] Direct impacts of exposure to Internet pornography include being upset or embarrassed; experiencing intrusion or harassment; and becoming stimulated or engaging in risky or inappropriate sexual activity.[25] Direct exposure to explicit sexual stimuli on the Internet can produce the type of premature erotic excitation described by Freud[30] in his explication of child sexual abuse trauma. Contemporary views of such effects provide insight into the origins of compulsive cybersex.

Children may become "sexually reactive" in response to cybersex exposure: engaging in compulsive masturbation, developing sexual variance, or perpetrating sexual aggression.[31-34] Greenfield[35] discussed the adverse developmental effects of participation in some adolescent chat rooms: disinhibition of sexual and aggressive behaviors, misinformation about sexuality and gender roles, and interpersonal irresponsibility. School counselors and youth workers have expressed concern that untreated sexual reactivity in children can lead to sexually variant and aggressive behavior.[36] Prior traumatization, social inadequacy, lack of intimacy, impulsivity, and lack of supervision or accountability characterize the process from victim to victimizer.[36,37] Children who have been sexually abused may molest other children, engage in delinquent conduct, or develop problems with compulsive sexual behavior.[38] Clearly the Internet sexual revolution has exacerbated risk for vulnerable children and adolescents.

Cybersex can produce problems in the workplace, as well. Approximately 70% of e-porn occurs on weekdays between 9:00 AM and 5:00 PM, the workday for many businesses and institutions.[5] Accessing sexual content on the Internet has become a significant issue for employers. In a large survey of 40,000 adults who use the Internet for sexual purposes,[39] 20% of respondents admitted to conducting online sexual activities at work. Two out of three companies have disciplined employees for "cyberslacking" or misusing the Internet at work, with 41% of the abuses involving pornography and 12% involving chatting.[40] Not only does online sexual activity contribute to loss of productivity and distraction from organizational goals, but cybersex can also violate policies and laws regarding privacy and other boundaries. Compulsive cybersex behavior in the workplace can contribute to a hostile work environment, sexual harassment, and cyberstalking.[41]

CASE STUDIES

The following case studies reflect how individuals can experience problems with compulsive cybersex behavior. Three case studies highlight the contribution of obsession, compulsion, and consequence[1] in the evolution of the problematic behavior. The cases also provide insight into potential treatment options. The following scenarios represent compilations of actual clinical cases encountered in practice. The names and other identifying information have been altered to preserve confidentiality.

Dan: Obsessive Preoccupation with Delicate Hair Cutting

Dan was a 35-year-old, white professional male married 7 years to Samantha, a 37-year-old woman with a 15-year-old daughter from a previous marriage. The couple presented for treatment of sexual dysfunction: low frequency of sexual outlet and erectile dysfunction secondary to delayed ejaculation. Dan had been avoiding sexual contact during the preceding 6 months because of increasing problems with maintaining an erection during intercourse. During individual and conjoint interviews, an underlying problem with compulsive cybersex was identified.

Dan revealed having a lifelong fetish involving a woman's long hair, which had evolved into his being obsessed with the delicate cutting of millimeters from long, blonde hair. As an adolescent, he shaped his preference by masturbating to fashion magazines depicting models with long, flowing hair. In adulthood, he indulged his sexual preoccupation by dating women with this "ideal" hair and touching or caressing the cherished object to become aroused and eventually ejaculate in consensual sexual activities. He was initially attracted to his wife due to her long "surfer girl" haircut and later surreptitiously indulged his fetish in their sex lives.

Over the years, he was attracted to Internet Web sites featuring long-haired models and celebrities, as well as commercial sites of hair salons and hair stylist supplies. These sites allowed him to indulge his vivid fantasy life and erotically stimulated him. By happenstance, he communicated with a like-minded individual, through a posting on a professional hair stylist Web site, who invited him to join an Internet hair-cutting fetish club. This quickly became his primary source for erotic exploration and stimulation, as well as his exclusive means for sexual arousal and outlet. He fantasized about the images and sounds on the fetish Web site to function sexually with his wife. When the fantasies failed or the novelty declined, he had difficulty maintaining his erection and ejaculating in marital intercourse.

Samantha disclosed that she had become increasingly aware of his special sexual preference during their courtship. Initially, she considered his attention to her hair as a compliment. Early in the marriage, she invited him to share his sexual fantasies with her. In subsequent marital sexual relations, she indulged, then tolerated, his fetish while encouraging him to expand the variety in their shared sexual life. After a few years, she wanted to cut her hair to a more contemporary style, but Dan strongly resisted her plan and encouraged her to bleach it to a lighter shade instead. They continued marital sexual relations on a less frequent basis until (unknown to her) Dan became obsessed with the fetish club and began to experience sexual dysfunction. Samantha became troubled when Dan repeatedly volunteered to trim not only her hair, but also the long hair of her daughter. Samantha later realized that her husband was in effect making sexual advances toward his stepdaughter. She confronted him in ongoing marital therapy.

This case study provides an excellent opportunity to understand the contribution of the Internet to the development of compulsive sexual behavior. Dan's fetish had developed before discovering the Internet hair salon and hair stylist industry Web sites. It rapidly evolved into a problematic obsession that interfered with the marital sexual relationship, however, under the influence of the powerful masturbatory conditioning associated with the online hair-cutting club. He not only masturbated to the sights and sounds in the club's Web site, but also received support and encouragement from other members for the alternative (and secretive) lifestyle. It was noteworthy that the most erotic or stimulating characteristic of the Web site that fueled his obsessive preoccupation with hair cutting, was a soundtrack of scissors snipping as they cut hair. This feature provided insight into how his symptom functioned and to implement treatment.

Initial treatment involved marital therapy to reduce conflicts and resentments associated with the sexless marriage and with Dan's various controlling maneuvers. Sex therapy based on the Masters and Johnson[42] model for treating erectile dysfunction and delayed ejaculation was then implemented. Dan's anxiety increased as he encountered opportunities for genuine intimacy. During a couple's session, he revealed that a paternal uncle had sexually abused him as a boy. He avoided disclosure because he loved his uncle, feared the information would hurt his father, and wondered if the abuse made him homosexual. While he could readily recall the abuse, he had dissociated feeling and meaning from his restrictive memories of the events. Dan experienced emotional release during the session as he described how his uncle, a barber, would touch the boy's penis under the drape while cutting his hair. Subsequently, the sound of hair cutting became the means for accessing recollections during Dan's exposure-based individual treatment for sexual abuse trauma.

After completing treatment for the sexual abuse, the power of the fetish diminished, although he continued to admire long hair as a symbol of his wife's feminine beauty. He was less anxious and better able to participate in the sex therapy homework assignments. The couple successfully completed sex therapy and enjoyed satisfying sexual outlet. During a brief follow-up visit, Samantha and Dan were able to address some power issues in their relationship culminating in her decision to cut her hair.

Dan's obsessive preoccupation with cybersex reenactment of childhood sexual abuse was consistent with Freud's[30,43] original accounts of psychic trauma and repetition compulsion. According to the central components of the Freudian model of trauma replay, premature or overexcitation of a child's vulnerable psychic system, especially when accompanied by betrayal of trust by the offending caregiver, drives the child to recreate the scene—actually or symbolically—to gain a sense of mastery or resolution.[44–48] Dan's cybersex obsessions originated in trauma replay and throughout his adult sexual life afforded him the means to avoid genuine intimacy while engaging in a semblance of sexual outlet with his partner at a safe emotional distance. The next case highlights how cybersex can function to express anger indirectly, manage stress, and ward off depression.

Anne: Compulsive Cybersex Engagement as Self-Treatment

Anne was a 25-year-old, single white female who was employed as a teacher in an urban elementary school. She grew up in an intact, conservatively religious home and participated actively in her church. From childhood to the present, Anne exhibited a wide range of symptoms of generalized anxiety and dysthymia, which she countered through overeating, perfectionism, and social withdrawal. She was an outstanding academic student and accomplished musician, but had few friendships, little social contact outside her church, and no dating experience. She attained academic honors and career gains in her field of elementary education.

Anne was also highly regarded for her work in the children's church and vacation Bible school. Although she became moderately obese in late adolescence, she experienced no other health problems. Anne's primary source of identity and life fulfillment related to being a teacher in the public school and church settings. She remained close to her parents and a younger sister, who was outgoing and prized for her beauty. Raised in a conflict-avoidant family, Anne lacked assertion skills and denied or minimized anger. When she was stressed or frustrated at work or when family or coworkers offended her, she redoubled her perfectionistic efforts by writing lesson plans or creating enrichment activities.

As a bright young woman who was technically proficient in educational media, Anne was attracted to computer-assisted instruction and applications of Internet Web sites in classroom teaching. By her senior year in college, however, Anne had used her laptop to discover the "dark side" of computer technology and Internet usage. She initially explored fantasy role-play game sites that provided controlled opportunities for disclosure and interaction with others. She especially enjoyed the role of a "wench" who could be ribald while receiving male attention that was sometimes rough or exploitative. While exploring role-playing, Anne began self-stimulation with devices she ordered through a sex toy Web site. She engaged daily in masturbation fueled by fantasies arising from game playing on the Internet. Although she did not recognize a pattern of use until later in therapy, Anne increased her masturbation to masochistic sexual fantasies during periods of high stress at work (eg, standardized testing days), when she felt especially empty and isolated, and after disagreements with significant others in which she predictably capitulated and apologized.

Anne's compulsive cybersex quickly progressed to cybering sessions with males she met online and to her disclosing extensive personal information to strangers met through chatting and social networking. Although ashamed of her secret sexual life, Anne was driven to continue the contacts and engage in cybersex-assisted masturbation, sometimes more than once daily and in settings such as the church restroom or an empty classroom. Her principal cautioned her about excessive computer use at school, which was contributing to a decline in her teaching performance. She withdrew into a sadomasochistic fantasy world and was forced to discontinue some of her church activities because she spent so many hours online.

Anne eventually initiated therapy for her compulsive cybersex behavior after some disturbing interactions with individuals she met online. Early in her descent into the fantasy world, she had given personal details and credit card information to someone she met online. That person then charged several thousand dollars in purchases. Anne was so ashamed of her secret life and embarrassed by her naiveté that she simply canceled the credit card without making a police report. The immediate precipitant for therapy involved personally meeting a man she had met online for a brief series of increasingly physically abusive and unsafe sexual contacts. One of the contacts involved his keeping her captive as a "sex slave" over a weekend.

This rapid progression from initial exploration to frequent and abusive sexual activities is characteristic of compulsive cybersex. The illusory cybersex world allowed Anne to compensate for social failures and to participate in a circumscribed form of sexual outlet. While she perceived control and victory in her role-play relationships, Anne realized she was increasingly out of control in a dangerous world populated by manipulative and exploitative persons. Her involvement in compulsive cybersex satisfied some recurring nonsexual functions: binding anxiety, overcoming emptiness and depressed mood, and turning anger inward through masochistic behavior.[48,49]

Anne's case is representative of female cybersex abusers in a clinical sample: relatively young, socially unskilled, excessive Internet users, compulsive overeaters, and depressed.[20] Her treatment involved referral to a psychiatrist for antidepressant medication, which also reduced her anxiety; participation in a faith-based program for sexual addiction treatment; brief solution-focused psychotherapy; attendance at an assertiveness training workshop for women; and participation in social networking offered by the singles' ministry of a nearby church. Anne realized treatment gains, maintained boundaries on Internet use, recovered her teaching excellence, and avoided relapse to maladaptive self-treatment of depression and anxiety. The significant consequences that she suffered heightened awareness of her problem and contributed to her decision to seek therapy before consequences became even more profound. The final case study represents the characteristic progression of compulsive cybersex toward harmful, life-altering consequences.

Joe: Profound Consequences Associated with Compulsive Cybersex

Joe was a 39-year-old white, married male, who was employed as a high school teacher in an affluent suburban school district. He was active in sponsoring student organizations and community groups devoted to the successful transition of students from school to college or work. He described his marriage of 14 years as satisfying, although the couple had been unable to have children and suffered two miscarriages in a 4-year period. Joe's attorney referred him to therapy for assessment and treatment of compulsive cybersex involving child pornography.

Joe was talented in science and technology, enjoying computer applications in education as well as personal use of the Internet at home. During the intake assessment, Joe acknowledged spending an average of 25 hours per week on the Internet in activities not related to work. Typically, he would spend hours online during late night "binges" of compulsive cybersex involving pornography and chatting with "swingers" on adult social networking sites. While he had not arranged face-to-face meetings with Internet sexual partners, he fantasized about involving his wife in the swinging lifestyle. Once he registered for a lifestyle convention without his wife's knowledge but cancelled the reservation after the novelty of this fantasy eroded as a result of compulsive masturbation. Joe later reported that his compulsive cybersex was fueled by the novelty and illicit quality of the stimuli. He would become fascinated with certain types of online sexual content, engage in compulsive masturbation, experience reinforcement erosion, lose interest, and progress to the next domain of interest.

Many of his cybersex interests and the resulting Internet site targets appeared to be conditioned by chance and accidents. After his descent into Internet pornography, Joe discovered that many Web sites and news groups promised new, increasingly elicit and extreme experiences. For example, participation in a local chat room led to cybering with a woman who subsequently introduced him to swinger and lifestyle sites. Exploration of pornography began with adult magazine images of nude women, progressed to videos of "amateur" couples engaged in sexual activities, included examination of "bicurious" Web sites and personal advertisements, and culminated in illicit images of a wide range of sexual variance and deviance. Joe's time-consuming investment in cybersex was fueled by affordability, in that he visited only free sites, and lack of accountability, since he had withdrawn emotionally from his marriage and his wife did not seem bothered by his late-night Internet sessions. His involvement in cybersex was guided by "pop-ups," e-mail invitations, chat room referrals, and other opportunistic ventures into new and exciting domains.

Joe was referred for therapy after being arrested for viewing child pornography, which remained in temporary files on the hard drive of his computer. Joe was shocked when local and federal law enforcement agents confronted him at his high school, confiscated his work (and later personal) computers, and interviewed him at the county jail. He was identified as a child pornographer and potential sex offender by evidence gathered through an explicit Web site, which served as a "sting" operation by law enforcement. Such proactive law enforcement efforts have contributed to a large number of arrests for Internet sex crimes against children.[50] Subsequently, Joe was arrested and charged with possession and conspiracy to distribute child pornography.

The consequences of Joe's conditioning to pursue increasingly deviant materials on the Internet resulted in his venturing into child pornography (accessed through invitations to view "teenage virgins" and "underage girls"). Joe's case did not fit the characteristics of a child pornographer or pedophile; however, participation in the objectification of children and deviant arousal conditioning could shape him toward hands-on offending.[51,52] Although he was remorseful, and psychosexual evaluation failed to identify pedophilia, compulsive cybersex resulted in loss of employment, marital separation, threat of divorce, loss of teaching credentials, shame, and potential incarceration. Given the limited extent of his involvement in child pornography and the court's perspective on his case, Joe was placed on probation and ordered to participate in therapy for compulsive cybersex. In many jurisdictions, mandatory prison sentences have been imposed for those caught in the "dark side of the net." Later Joe and his wife were able to restore their marriage by participating in integrative marital and sexual therapy after careful disclosure of secrets and ongoing attendance in the Sex Addicts Anonymous self-help group.[53–55]

These three case studies offer details of the pathogenesis of compulsive cybersex. The case of Dan emphasized the role of obsession or preoccupation in the development of a paraphilia through trauma replay. Anne's case represented dependence on compulsive behavior to self-manage depression and anxiety. Her case included gender issues, including risks involved in personally meeting online partners. The final case study highlighted the profound consequences associated with compulsive cybersex. Based on individual sexual behavior conditioning and dysfunctional marital dynamics, Joe and his wife faced overwhelming loss and chaos by virtue of his descent into compulsive cybersex. The case studies presented compulsive cybersex in terms of obsession, compulsion, and consequence. Additional functions, dynamics, and characteristics should be taken into consideration in clinical judgment and treatment planning.

TREATMENT APPROACHES

Treatment of compulsive cybersex is based on the function of the problematic behavior in the lives of the patient and significant others. Typically, an individual seeks treatment after disclosure of online sexual activities, frequently after consequences have accumulated. Occasionally, compulsive cybersex is discovered in the course of intake evaluation or treatment for another disorder or relationship problem. Some couples seek therapy for sexual dysfunction or dissatisfaction in which cybersex interferes with normal sexual function. Individuals presenting with substance use disorders and other process addictions, such as pathological gambling or eating disorder, may reveal a concurrent problem with compulsive cybersex. Many compulsive cybersex patients present comorbid anxiety and affective disorders. The presentation and function of compulsive cybersex determine the initial context of treatment.

Typologies have been offered to organize treatment planning. Several contributors characterized compulsive cybersex as a form of sexual addiction in which users engage in a predictable cycle leading to powerlessness and unmanageability.[5,6] The cycle of cybersex addiction progresses through four steps: preoccupation, ritualization, compulsive sexual behavior, and unmanageability and despair.[5] Cybersex user categories included *appropriate recreational users*, who engage in online sexual activities without problems or consequences; *inappropriate recreational users*, who are not compulsive, but introduce cybersex content in improper situations (eg, at work); *discovery group* of individuals for whom Internet stimuli trigger fantasies, preoccupations, and compulsions (eg, sexually reactive or primed children); *predisposed group* of persons who have been struggling with sexual issues or problems; and *lifelong sexual compulsives* who experience increasing symptoms of addiction to cybersex.[5] Other typologies do not necessarily embrace addiction as an explanatory model and tend to emphasize other functions and dynamics.

Another typology of compulsive cybersex patients explored gender differences, as well as loner and paraphiliac subtypes.[20] This study explored characteristics of persons who sought treatment for compulsive cybersex. In the clinical sample, males were older than female users and more likely to be chemically dependent, sexually addicted, and involved in the Twelve-Step recovery community. Female cybersex abusers were similar to nonproblematic users of the Internet and more likely to present symptoms of posttraumatic stress disorder (PTSD) and either compulsive overeating or bulimia. Both groups presented symptoms of depression and used the Internet to pursue self-reported interests in paraphilias, romance/dating, and swinging. Some cybersex abusers in the study developed problematic use because they were essentially loners: socially unskilled men and isolative, obese women. A subset of socially isolative users presented strong paraphilias, fueled by masturbatory conditioning of variant sexual preferences.[31,56] Other authors emphasized the role of the Internet as society's new red-light district in the etiology of paraphilias, including pedophilia.[57]

The typologies of compulsive cybersex afford some insight into the underlying dynamics and functions that should be addressed in intake, assessment, and treatment planning. Among paraphiliac and exploitative patients, some individuals will present criminal histories and pending legal consequences that complicate the evaluation process. Some of these patients may be mandated to participate in treatment as a condition of diversion, probation, or parole. Similarly, employee assistance programs may require ongoing treatment and progress reports for workers who have violated boundaries and policies through compulsive cybersex behaviors. Many voluntary patients face potentially life-altering consequences, such as loss of one's marriage or professional privileges, which compel them to become involved in treatment. Most compulsive cybersex patients tend to underestimate the severity of their problems, engaging in considerable denial and minimization. To enhance insight and motivation for treatment compliance, it would be helpful to engage the patient in exploration of the motives, dynamics, and functions of their problematic behaviors.

Compulsive cybersex can be conceptualized as maladaptive coping, conditioned behavior, dissociative reenactment of life trauma, courtship disorder, intimacy dysfunction, and addictive behavior. Compulsive cybersex functions as maladaptive coping when the problematic behavior represents an attempt to manage stress or reduce anxiety; ward off boredom, loneliness, or depression; express frustration and anger directly or indirectly; and bolster a fragile ego.[10,20] Comorbid clinical syndromes, especially anxiety and affective disorders, may need to be addressed through psychotropic medication management and development of effective coping strategies such as systematic muscle relaxation.[57,58] Among heavy, long-term Internet users, depression and substance use disorders (especially alcoholism) may demand initial attention, while suicidality is a risk among younger, recent-onset "binge" users.[8] Regardless of the initial presentation, psychiatric evaluation and psychotropic medication should be considered early in the clinical judgment process. Some cybersex-based paraphilias, hypersexuality, and offender behaviors can be managed through pharmacological treatment involving antipsychotic, antidepressant, and anti-androgenic medications.[16,57]

The conditioning process in compulsive cybersex accounts for the development of particular preferences, as well as the progression of the behaviors over time. Although research data are equivocal, there is evidence that sexual arousal may be affected through classical conditioning, leading to variant interests and paraphilias in some cases.[59–61] In addition, sexual behavior is subject to operant conditioning in which the near future occurrence of a problematic behavior can increase through the powerful reinforcement afforded by masturbation to orgasm.[61,62] Therefore, some compulsive cybersex behaviors, especially paraphilias, may require laboratory-based assessment of sexual arousal (eg, penile plethysmography), sexual arousal reconditioning (eg, olfactory aversion and covert sensitization), and other cognitive-behavioral treatments.[63–67] Conditioning of compulsive cybersex behaviors tends to occur along a developmental trajectory, frequently determined by early life experiences.

Some confusing and abusive life experiences contribute to conditioning of compulsive cybersex by functioning as dissociative reenactment of life trauma. The case study of Dan's paraphiliac cybersex revealed the origins in his childhood sexual abuse that culminated in a preoccupation that held the code for trauma resolution. When cybersex involves dissociative reenactment, treatment for the underlying life trauma is indicated. Most interventions for survivors of trauma involve some counterconditioning and self-efficacy enhancement by means of exposure to the traumatic stimuli.[68,69] In addition, the most dissociative patients benefit from therapy designed to access split-off parts or ego states, improve internal communication in the self-system, resolve conflicts, and decrease self-injurious and sabotaging maneuvers.[48,70–72] Hypnosis,[73] ego states therapy,[74] internal family systems therapy,[75] and voice therapy[76] can produce beneficial outcomes for dissociative compulsive cybersex patients. Therapy for dissociative cybersex states not only reduces or eliminates the compulsion, but also advances the ego strength and interpersonal development of the patient.

Compulsive cybersex is fundamentally a courtship disorder in which development of the normally integrative function of sexuality in the mature adult is disrupted, distorted, or displaced. Money[77] was the first to describe comprehensively the development of lovemaps that organize sexual information processing and decision making. Classically, courtship behavior was determined by sexual attractivity, proceptivity, and receptivity in partners leading to mate selection, sexual outlet, conception, birth, and child rearing.[78] Compulsive cybersex evidences displacement, omission, inclusion, transposition, and other distortions of underlying lovemaps such that normal courtship behavior is disrupted. Money[77] identified the following distorted lovemaps: sacrifice and expiation, marauding and predation, mercantile and venal strategies, fetishes and talismans, stigmata and eligibility, and solicitation and allure. Contemporary models have asserted that sexual schemas guide and regulate behavior.[79,80] Sexual self-schemas, including implicit self-talk and imagery, must be modified in the course of therapy to overcome problematic biases and make room for an intimacy-enhancing sexual relationship with a consenting adult partner. Treatment for distorted lovemaps and dysfunctional self-schemas involves relational therapies such as group psychotherapy and marital and sexual therapy.

Intimacy enhancement is the outcome of sexuality guided by healthy lovemaps or self-schemas. While the array of acceptable sexual behaviors for an intimate couple may be large, healthy sexual outlet increases intimacy in a committed relationship. Intimate sexuality is partner-oriented: heightening the capacity for physical and emotional closeness in the romantic couple. Compulsive cybersex contributes to the violation of relational boundaries and results in injuries such as feeling violated or betrayed. Cybersex causes intimacy dysfunction when the online sexual activity alienates a person from a healthy relationship with oneself and one's partner. Treatment of intimacy dysfunction should include a couple in the safe haven or *holding environment* of interventions that address bonding, attachment, and closeness.[81] Effective therapies for intimacy enhancement are relationship or systems-oriented and integrate sex and marital therapy to promote good object relations or psychosexual health.[42,82,83]

The final domain of comprehensive treatment of compulsive cybersex addresses addictive behavior. Compulsive cybersex can progress until it evidences the powerlessness and unmanageability associated with addiction. Compulsive cybersex may be manifested in a more pervasive addictive lifestyle in which the patient presents with alcoholism, chemical dependence, eating disorder, pathological gambling, or another addictive behavior. When multiple addictions occur in an addictive lifestyle, the most important issue is determining if the patient would benefit from outpatient services or requires more intensive, stabilizing treatment in a hospital or residential treatment center. A related issue is whether an addictive patient will comply with a medication regimen or another intervention.

A recurring issue in treating compulsive cybersex is *relapse prevention*. Structure, intensity, and pacing of treatment interventions can affect risk of relapse. Generally, it is advisable to implement relapse prevention methods at the outset of any treatment protocol. The classic model of Marlatt and Gordon,[84] involving cognitive and behavioral interventions, can be introduced in a psychoeducational group and strengthened through homework. Related to relapse prevention is the transtheoretical model of the stages of change,[85,86] which highlights treatment tasks during a predictable sequence of events: precontemplation, contemplation, preparation, action, maintenance, and termination. Some addictionologists believe that sexual addicts should participate in lifelong recovery by regularly attending Twelve-Step groups such as Sex Addicts Anonymous. Participation in ongoing recovery groups provides opportunities for relapse prevention, social support, and spiritual development.

Comprehensive treatment involves implementing an individually tailored treatment package that addresses the major functions, dynamics, motives, and characteristics of the particular patient presenting compulsive cybersex. The components of treatment include relapse prevention, intimacy enhancement, lovemap reconstruction, dissociative states therapy, arousal reconditioning, and coping skills training. Initially, the patient should refrain from using the Internet, although computer usage with sufficient boundary and accountability is a treatment goal. Decisions about level of care and medication are made early in treatment in conjunction with group approaches for relapse prevention. Intensive individual therapy should be implemented in preparation for marital and sexual therapy. Participation in an ongoing recovery group not only enhances the motivation for change, but also prepares the individual to find meaning within healthy relationships.

SUMMARY

Compulsive cybersex has become a significant problem for many men and women who have fallen prey to the accessibility, affordability, and anonymity of online sexual behaviors. Some patients develop problems with compulsive cybersex due to predisposition or accidental conditioning experiences. Other compulsive users of cybersex present with underlying trauma, depression, or addiction. Three case studies highlighted obsession, compulsion, and consequence in the pathogenesis of compulsive cybersex. While men and women differ somewhat in their use of cybersex, both genders exhibit maladaptive coping, conditioned behavior, dissociative reenactment of life trauma, courtship disorder, intimacy dysfunction, and addictive behavior. Comprehensive treatment of compulsive cybersex would include the following components: relapse prevention, intimacy enhancement, lovemap reconstruction, dissociative states therapy, arousal reconditioning, and coping skills training. Thanks to recent treatment advances in several fields, help is available for those caught in the dark side of the net.

REFERENCES

1. Cooper A, Delmonico DL, Griffin-Shelley E, et al. Online sexual activity: an examination of potentially problematic behaviors. Sexual Addiction & Compulsivity 2004;11:129–43.
2. Daneback K, Cooper A, Mansson SA. An Internet study of cybersex participants. Arch Sex Behav 2005;34:321–8.
3. Ross MW. Typing, doing, and being: sexuality and the Internet. J Sex Res 2005; 42:342–52.
4. Cooper A. Online sexual activity in the new millennium. Contemp Sex 2004;38(3): i–vii.
5. Carnes P, Delmonico DL, Griffin E. In the shadows of the net: breaking free of compulsive online sexual behavior. Center City (MN): Hazelden; 2001.
6. Schneider J, Weiss R. Cybersex exposed: simple fantasy or obsession. Center City (MN): Hazelden; 2001.
7. Cooper A, Scherer CR, Boies SC, et al. Sexuality on the Internet: from sexual exploration to pathological expression. Prof Psychol Res Pr 1999;30:154–64.
8. Mathy RM, Cooper A. The duration and frequency of Internet use in a nonclinical sample: suicidality, behavioral problems, and treatment histories. Psychother Theor Res Pract Train 2003;40:125–35.
9. Mitchell KJ, Becker-Blease KA, Finkelhor D. Inventory of problematic Internet experiences encountered in clinical practice. Prof Psychol Res Pr 2005;36:498–509.
10. Nichols LA, Nicki R. Development of a psychometrically sound Internet addiction scale: a preliminary step. Psychol Addict Behav 2004;18:381–4.
11. Young KS. Internet addiction: a new clinical phenomenon and its consequences. Am Behav Sci 2004;48:402–15.
12. Kibby M, Costello B. Between the image and the act: interactive sex entertainment on the Internet. Sexualities 2001;4:353–69.
13. Lillie JJM. Cyberporn, sexuality, and the net apparatus. Convergence 2004;10: 43–65.
14. Whitty WT. Cyber-flirting: playing at love on the Internet. Theory Psychol 2003;13: 339–57.
15. Hertlein KM, Piercy FP. Internet infidelity: a critical review of the literature. The Family Journal: Counseling and Therapy for Couples and Families 2006;14:366–71.
16. Kafka MP. Sex offending and sexual appetite: the clinical and theoretical relevance of hypersexual desire. Int J Offender Ther Comp Criminol 2003;47:439–51.
17. Cooper A, Galbreath N, Becker MA. Sex on the Internet: furthering our understanding of men with online sexual problems. Psychol Addict Behav 2004;18: 223–30.
18. Kuipers G. The social construction of digital danger: debating, defusing, and inflating the moral dangers of online humor and pornography in the Netherlands and the United States. New Media Soc 2006;8:379–400.

19. Cooper A. The Internet and sexuality: into the new millennium. J Sex Educ Ther 1997;22:5–6.
20. Schwartz MF, Southern S. Compulsive cybersex: the new tea room. In: Cooper A, editor. Cybersex: the dark side of the force: a special issue of the journal Sexual Addiction & Compulsivity. New York: Routledge; 2000. p. 127–44.
21. Delmonico DL, Griffin EJ, Moriarty J. Cybersex unhooked: a workbook for breaking free from compulsive online sexual behavior. Center City (MN): Hazelden; 2001.
22. Stoller R. Perversion: the erotic form of hatred. New York: Pantheon Books; 1975.
23. Cooper A, Delmonico DL, Burg R. Cybersex users, abusers, and compulsives: new findings and implications. Sexual Addiction & Compulsivity 2000;7:5–29.
24. Leiblum S, Doring N. Internet sexuality: known risks and fresh chances for women. In: Cooper A, editor. Sex & the Internet: a guidebook for clinicians. New York: Routledge; 2002. p. 19–45.
25. Ybarra ML, Mitchell KJ. Exposure to Internet pornography among children and adolescents: a national survey. Cyberpsychol Behav 2005;8:473–86.
26. Mitchell KJ, Finkelhor D, Wolak J. Victimization of youths on the Internet. Journal of Aggression, Maltreatment & Trauma 2003;8(1-2):1–39.
27. Mitchell KJ, Wolak J, Finkelhor D. Trends in youth reports of sexual solicitations, harassment and unwanted exposure to pornography on the Internet. J Adolesc Health 2007;40:116–26.
28. Manning JC. The impact of Internet pornography on marriage and the family: a review of research. Sexual Addiction & Compulsivity 2006;13:131–65.
29. Schneider JP. The new "elephant in the living room": effects of compulsive cybersex behaviors on the spouse. In: Cooper A, editor. Sex & the Internet: a guidebook for clinicians. New York: Routledge; 2002. p. 169–86.
30. Freud S. On the aetiology of hysteria. In: Strachey J, editor, The standard edition of the complete psychological works of Sigmund Freud, vol. 3. London: Hogarth Press; 1962. p. 189–221.
31. Freeman-Longo RE. Children, teens, and sex on the Internet. Sexual Addiction & Compulsivity 2000;7:75–90.
32. Longo RE, Brown SM, Price Orcutt D. Effects of Internet sexuality on children and adolescents. In: Cooper A, editor. Sex on the Internet: a guidebook for clinicians. New York: Brunner/Routledge; 2002. p. 87–108.
33. Malamuth NM, Addison T, Koss M. Pornography and sexual aggression: are there reliable effects and can we understand them? Annu Rev Sex Res 2000; 11:26–94.
34. Zilman D. Influence of unrestrained access to erotica on adolescents' and young adults' dispositions toward sexuality. J Adolesc Health 2000;27:41–4.
35. Greenfield PM. Inadvertent exposure to pornography on the Internet: implications for peer-to-peer file sharing networks for child development and families. J Appl Dev Psychol 2004;25:741–50.
36. Cashwell CS, Bloss KK, McFarland JE. From victim to client: preventing the cycle of sexual reactivity. School Counselor 1995;42:233–8.
37. Rasmussen LA, Burton JE, Christopherson BJ. Precursors to offending and the trauma outcome process in sexually reactive children. J Child Sex Abus 1992; 1(1):33–48.
38. Johnson TC. Some considerations about sexual abuse and children with sexual behavioral problems. Journal of Trauma & Dissociation 2002;3:83–105.
39. Cooper A, Scherer C, Mathy R. Overcoming methodological concerns in the investigation of online sexual activities. Cyberpsychol Behav 2001;4:437–48.

40. Greenfield DN. Virtual addiction: help for netheads, cyberfreaks, and those who love them. Oakland (CA): New Harbinger; 1999.
41. Cooper A, McLoughlin I, Reich P, et al. Virtual sexuality in the workplace: a wake-up call for clinicians, employers, and employees. In: Cooper A, editor. Sex & the Internet: a guidebook for clinicians. New York: Routledge; 2002. p. 109–28.
42. Masters WH, Johnson VE. Human sexual inadequacy. Boston: Little, Brown & Company; 1970.
43. Freud S. Recollecting, repeating, and working through. In: Strachey J, editor and translator. The standard edition of the complete psychological works of Sigmund Freud, vol. 12. London: Hogarth Press; 1958. p. 145–56.
44. Chu JA. The repetition compulsion revisited: reliving dissociated trauma. Psychotherapy 1991;28:327–32.
45. Hall JM. Dissociative experiences of women child abuse survivors: a selective constructivist review. Trauma Violence Abuse 2003;4:283–308.
46. Kirman NF. The repetition compulsion revisited. Issues Psychoanal Psychol 1996; 18:36–49.
47. Marcel M. Freud's traumatic memory: reclaiming seduction theory and revisiting Oedipus. Pittsburgh (PA): Duquesne University Press; 2005.
48. Southern S. The tie that binds: sadomasochism in female addicted trauma survivors. Sexual Addiction & Compulsivity 2002;9:209–29.
49. Baumeister RF. Escaping the self: alcoholism, spirituality, masochism, and other flights from the burden of selfhood. New York: Basic Books; 1991.
50. Mitchell KJ, Wolak J, Finkelhor D. Police posing as juveniles online to catch sex offenders: is it working? Sex Abuse 2005;17:241–67.
51. Quayle E, Taylor M. Child pornography and the internet: perpetuating a cycle of abuse. Deviant Behav 2002;23:331–62.
52. Quayle E, Taylor M. Model of problematic internet use in people with sexual interest in children. Cyberpsychol Behav 2003;6:93–106.
53. Corley MD, Schneider JP. Disclosing secrets: when, to whom & how much to reveal. Wickenburg (AZ): Gentle Path Press; 2002.
54. Schwartz MF, Masters WH. Inhibited sexual desire: the Master and Johnson Institute treatment model. In: Leiblum SR, Rosen RC, editors. Sexual desire disorders. New York: Guilford Press; 1988. p. 229–42.
55. Schnarch DM. Desire problems: a systemic perspective. In: Leiblum SR, Rosen RC, editors. Principles and practice of sex therapy. 3rd edition. New York: Guilford Press; 2000. p. 17–56.
56. Lamb M. Cybersex: research notes on the characteristics of visitors to online chat rooms. Deviant Behav 1998;19:121–35.
57. Galbreath NW, Berlin FS, Sawyer D. Paraphilias and the Internet. In: Cooper A, editor. Sex & the Internet: a guidebook for clinicians. New York: Routledge; 2002. p. 187–205.
58. Delmonico DL, Griffin E, Carnes PJ. Treating online compulsive sexual behavior: when cybersex is the drug of choice. In: Cooper A, editor. Sex & the Internet: a guidebook for clinicians. New York: Routledge; 2002. p. 147–67.
59. Hoffman H, Janssen E, Turner L. Classical conditioning of sexual arousal in women and men: effects of varying awareness and biological relevance of the conditioned stimulus. Arch Sex Behav 2004;33:43–53.
60. Letourneau EJ, O'Donohue W. Classical conditioning of female sexual arousal. Arch Sex Behav 1997;26:63–78.
61. Plaud JJ, Martini JR. The respondent conditioning of male sexual arousal. Behav Modif 1999;23:254–68.

62. Pfaus JG, Kippin TE, Centeno S. Conditioning and sexual behavior: a review. Horm Behav 2001;40:291–321.
63. Marshall WL. Assessment, treatment, and theorizing about sex offenders: developments during the past twenty years and future directions. Crim Justice Behav 1996;23:162–99.
64. Maletzky BM, Steinhauser C. A 25-year follow-up of cognitive/behavioral therapy with 7,275 sexual offenders. Behav Modif 2002;26:123–47.
65. Schwartz BK. Effective treatment techniques for sex offenders. Psychiatr Ann 1992;22:315–9.
66. Wiederman MW. Paraphilia and fetishism. The Family Journal: Counseling and Therapy for Couples and Families 2003;11:315–21.
67. Witt P, Sager W. Procedures for treating deviant sexual arousal patterns. In: Keller PA, Heyman SR, editors. Innovations in clinical practice: a source book, vol. 7. Sarasota (FL): Professional Resource Exchange; 1988. p. 89–98.
68. Keane TM, Albano AM, Blake DD. Current trends in the treatment of post-traumatic stress symptoms. In: Basoglu M, editor. Torture and its consequences: current treatment approaches. New York: Cambridge University Press; 1992. p. 363–401.
69. Saigh PA. Effects of flooding on memories of patients with posttraumatic stress disorder. In: Douglas JD, Marmar CR, editors. Trauma, memory, and dissociation. Washington, DC: American Psychiatric Association; 1998. p. 285–320.
70. Schwartz MF. Reenactment related to bonding and hypersexuality. Sexual Addiction & Compulsivity 1996;3:195–212.
71. Schwartz MF, Galperin LD, Masters WH. Dissociation and treatment of compulsive reenactment of trauma: sexual compulsivity. In: Hunter M, editor. Adult survivors of sexual abuse: treatment innovations. Thousand Oaks (CA): Sage; 1995. p. 42–55.
72. Schwartz MF, Southern S. Manifestations of damaged development of the human affectional systems and developmentally based psychotherapies. Sexual Addiction & Compulsivity 1999;6:163–75.
73. Yapko MD. Trancework: an introduction to the practice of clinical hypnosis. 2nd edition. New York: Brunner/Mazel; 1990.
74. Watkins JG, Watkins HH. Ego states: theory and therapy. New York: W.W. Norton; 1997.
75. Schwartz RC. Internal family systems therapy. New York: Guilford Press; 1995.
76. Firestone RW, Firestone L, Catlett J. Sex and love in intimate relationships. Washington, DC: American Psychological Association; 2006.
77. Money J. Lovemaps: clinical concepts of sexual/erotic health and pathology, paraphilia, and gender transposition in childhood, adolescence, and maturity. New York: Irvington Publishers; 1986.
78. Beach FA. Sexual attractivity, proceptivity, and receptivity in female mammals. Horm Behav 1976;7:105–38.
79. Anderson BL, Cyranowski JM, Espindle D. Men's sexual self-schema. J Pers Soc Psychol 1999;76:645–61.
80. Cyranowski JM, Anderson BL. Schemas, sexuality, and romantic attachment. J Pers Soc Psychol 1998;74:1364–79.
81. Winnicott DW. The maturational process and the facilitating environment. New York: International Universities Press; 1965.
82. Kaplan HS. The new sex therapy: active treatment of sexual dysfunctions. New York: Brunner/Mazel; 1974.
83. Schnarch DM. Constructing the sexual crucible: an integration of sexual and marital therapy. New York: Norton; 1991.

84. Marlatt GA, Gordon JR. Relapse prevention: maintenance strategies in the treatment of addictive behaviors. New York: Guilford Press; 1985.
85. Prochaska JO, DiClemente CC, Norcross JC. In search of how people change: applications to addictive behaviors. Am Psychol 1992;47:1102–14.
86. Prochaska JO, Norcross JC. Stages of change. Psychotherapy 2001;38:443–8.

Female Sexual Compulsivity: a New Syndrome

Martha Turner, MD

KEYWORDS

- Female sexual compulsivity • Childhood sexual abuse
- Addiction • Sex • Masturbation

Because of its secretiveness, sexual compulsivity is not as obvious a problem as alcohol or drug abuse, although it is just as lethal.[1] It often begins in childhood and flourishes in adolescence, before the emergence of substance abuse. Family histories generally reflect issues such as little real intimacy, inconsistent rules, inadequate supervision, too high or low expectations, and histories of addictions that may date back generations. In these families, children are often neglected, mistreated, or exploited, rendering them vulnerable to sexual and other kinds of abuse by those within or outside of the family. They may, inadvertently, discover behaviors such as masturbation and fantasy/imaginary relationships, and other nonsexual behaviors, such as food, to cope with the physical and emotional distress over their powerlessness and limited choices. Whatever escape provides the greatest rush away from psychic pain and promotes survival will be used repeatedly until it takes on a life of its own.

Possibly 4 of 10 adults in United States culture may be sexually compulsive.[2] Although most sexual compulsives are men, increasing numbers of women are also exploring novel forms of sexual behaviors, especially on the Internet. The illusion of feeling safe (because it occurs in their homes), along with the availability, anonymity, and low cost, encourage many women to become addicted to cybersex. Imagination and adventure create feelings of arousal and power that seem limitless.[3,4] Internet intrigue, however, can lead to sexual encounters outside the home with potentially tragic outcomes. Without the advantage of social and visual cues, information obtained only from the computer, and later the telephone, severely limits women in their ability to accurately determine the outcome of meeting an Internet acquaintance face-to-face. The intensity and excitement draw them away from their reality and responsibilities and can seriously cloud judgment.

In recent studies of cybersex, 1% of people had serious problems with sex on the Internet, with 40% of these women. Some women seem not to have a background of trauma and would never have ventured out of the home for encounters, except for the compelling sense of power they felt online.[3] This consequence is not unlike the effects

Private Practice, Bryn Mawr, PA, USA
E-mail address: mtshrink@aol.com

Psychiatr Clin N Am 31 (2008) 713–727
doi:10.1016/j.psc.2008.06.004
0193-953X/08/$ – see front matter © 2008 Elsevier Inc. All rights reserved.

psych.theclinics.com

of cocaine in the 1980s when recreational use led to a rapid escalation and tragic consequences. Most women who have serious cybersex problems, however, have histories of significant trauma.

Sexual compulsivity is uniquely insidious; it starts earlier in life and lasts longer than most other compulsive behaviors, such as alcoholism, before it is addressed. For many, sex may be the primary behavior of choice. Drugs, alcohol, and food are secondary and often used to augment sexual fantasy or activity and coping with the aftermath of despair. Crossing and substituting compulsive behaviors are common. For example, when one stops drinking or binge eating, sexual behaviors may escalate. Secondary compulsions are often treated first, because they are more obvious and more socially acceptable to treat than sexual compulsivity. In facilities that treat only chemical addictions, undiagnosed sexual compulsivity or other compulsive behaviors, such as gambling (video poker is currently very popular among women) and eating, are often factors in recidivism.

Although longing to be loved and feel normal, female sexual compulsives have developed skewed thinking about love that translates into wanting power and control over others (usually men). The need to prevail in adult relationships results from profound powerlessness experienced in childhood with subsequent immense amounts of shame. For example, in the 1977 movie "*Looking for Mr. Goodbar*",[5] the woman protagonist is a schoolteacher of deaf children by day and cruises bars by night. She experienced a disabling medical disorder as a child and then turned her original helplessness into being a powerful sexual seductress as an adult. Her sexual behavior progresses. She combines alcohol and drugs with sexual acting out, becoming increasingly less discriminating of the men she chooses for encounters. Tragically, a stranger she chooses as a sexual partner murders her.

Generally, the sexual compulsive uses her behavior as a main coping mechanism, often unaware of its conscious connection to childhood events. Although masturbation and fantasy may have saved the sanity of the young person, her progression to extensive sexual behaviors becomes seriously maladaptive in adulthood, destroying and exploiting relationships as she organizes her life around fantasy or actual encounters. If she is in a relationship, her partner and children will experience neglect and other consequences as her disorder progresses.

CULTURAL CHALLENGES

Charlotte Kasl[6] has written extensively about women's ongoing search for love and power, describing the intertwining of compulsive sexuality and codependence (seeking security, being cared for, and being in charge while disregarding their own needs) as a typical style for women. In her later book, she is further convinced that compulsive sexuality in women is partly a reaction to oppression by our patriarchal culture. Oppression triggers the creation of addictions as a release from this oppression, while fostering rigid thinking and a sin/redemption mindset.

Patriarchy is a hierarchy in which women and other marginalized people are assigned a subordinate position to the dominant white male in United States culture. Some traits of patriarchy are conscious but many are unconscious, passed down for generations and distorted by myths of male superiority, expectations that needs will be met by the opposite sex, and the wounds experienced by both men and women from these beliefs.[7] Women are raised to be codependent, and therefore are taught to internalize this oppression (passivity, deferring to others, underachieving) so that patriarchy and capitalism can be maintained.

However, victims want to prevail. Women and minorities have been protesting this oppression in the past few decades, encountering much resistance as the hierarchy fights to keep the *status quo*. Victims are blamed (eg, women invite rape, the court system retraumatizes them), the land is destroyed (eg, war, overgrazing, overdeveloping), and women lose touch with nature's balance and harmony (eg, feminine energy) in the quest for material things (capitalism) while never feeling good enough (diminished self-esteem so women stay in their place). Finding one's place in American culture is even more difficult for lesbians.[8]

Compulsive sexual behavior for men has generally been more about objectifying sex (voyeurism, exhibitionism, anonymous, intrusive, trading, paying for sex, exploitive), whereas women's behaviors are more about seeking relationships and security (fantasy, seduction, and exhibitionism in wardrobe). These generalizations are not as distinct as they once were, and may reflect other changes in American culture, with previously typical roles for men and women blurring.

An extreme form of compulsive sexuality is sexual abuse of children. Men are usually perceived as the perpetrators and punished by removal from the home or incarceration. Women can also be perpetrators but are often not considered as threatening because they are seen as the caregivers and protectors of children. Sexual abuse by women is often viewed as the woman being an accomplice to the male perpetrator, on whom she depends, rather than the prime initiator; women are coerced by these men to participate to avoid being abandoned. Tragically, most of these women were themselves sexually abused in childhood, usually by a male family member.

A smaller group of women, who sexually abuse children without male coercion, were sexually abused before the age of 10 years and are more seriously mentally disturbed, usually having no partners. They are also less coercive than women who abuse with a male accomplice, tending to use games to seduce the children they abuse, and probably identifying with them.

A major contributing factor in women who sexually abuse children is the mother–daughter attachment. Girls learn their female identity from their mothers. If they don't have enough consistent nurturance, they fail to develop a sense of self. They will feel lost and worthless, needing others to confirm and approve of who they are. Our culture supports this dependency and inferiority. Protesting is discouraged in girls. Depression and anger ensue, finding expression later in behavior. Women sex offenders more frequently choose same-sex victims (daughters), seeing themselves in the girls they offend and projecting onto them the displaced anger they have at their own mothers for their plight in society. They do not pursue sex, as men usually do, but the attachment and nurturing they did not receive in childhood. Without secure attachment bonds, girls cannot differentiate from their mothers and are consequently unable to become independent, self-sufficient women who can make conscious choices about their lives.[9]

DIAGNOSING

One problem in diagnosing sexual compulsivity is that it can present clinically like other psychiatric disorders, such as anxiety, depression, bipolar disorder, sociopathy, narcissism, obsessive–compulsive disorder, alcoholism, posttraumatic stress disorder (PTSD), and other personality disorders. In fact, many psychiatric disorders may co-exist with sexual compulsivity, so that the diagnosis is complicated.

Sexual compulsivity is finally diagnosed, order emerges from the chaos and a clear direction for treatment is possible. Therapists must be empathetic and nonjudgmental when taking a thorough history. Questions must be asked about excessive preoccupation, behaviors, and consequences concerning the patient's sexual activities. A Sexual Addiction Screening Test for women is available online (www.sexhelp.com). The questions address relationship disturbance, preoccupation/loss of control, and degrading/shameful feelings. The patient may not disclose or even recognize any sexually offending behavior. Because of the enormous amount of shame women sexual compulsives experience (women are deemed guardians of their morality), patients may be more comfortable and candid filling out a questionnaire privately rather than with a therapist.

TREATMENT

Patients will resist treatment because of their shame and the terror of giving up a dependable coping mechanism and source of power. Deception, lying, denial, and manipulation are common traits of this disorder. To begin a therapeutic relationship, therapists must provide and have boundaries that are strong and consistent. Therapists also need to know their own sexual issues and keep them in check. One small indication of judgment or vicarious interest in a woman's behaviors may result either in the patient leaving therapy (physically or through dissociation) or sensing that she is being encouraged to be seductive, thus repeating old patterns. Initially, patients will not be able to reveal their entire history because they have been carrying secrets that defy the cultural norms for women and are reluctant to reveal them. It may take years before patients can disclose the worst of them to a therapist. For example, sadomasochism in women are most likely reenactments of their trauma, and may not have been shared before.[7] Meanwhile, the therapist can begin addressing the more destructive behaviors the patient has been able to admit.

Chemical dependencies are more acceptable disorders than sexual ones, and must be arrested for patients to be cognitively available in treatment. Patients may find other compulsive experiences or behaviors to replace the ones they know they must stop. Medications may be used to help stabilize intense anxiety and depression when beginning recovery. Therapists must understand how raw and terrified patients feel in giving up what has worked for years.

Support groups specific to sexually compulsive women are invaluable. The 12 steps can be very useful and cost-effective for maintaining sobriety. These meetings, however, continue to emphasize obedience, humility (often becoming humiliating), and a rather immature (turn it over) spirituality, which tends to perpetuate the oppression women have always felt. Women have an enormous need to belong, be accepted as they are (not as sex objects), be encouraged to question, make choices that work for them, and feel empowered.

At mixed 12-step meetings, veterans in the meetings often prey on women just beginning recovery, who then feel unsafe and leave or become involved romantically so early that their personal work is stalled and nothing changes. Sponsors can be so rigid that, if their direction is not followed, the person sponsored may be rejected for having resistance or questions. Women entering a 12-step program for the first time are vulnerable and do not have healthy defenses or the clarity to make good decisions.

Women for Sobriety and other women's groups are probably better suited for recovery as long as respect, gentleness, encouragement to be responsible for one's self, increased awareness, and self-reliance are the standards. Women can also perpetuate the oppression on each other because that was how they were raised.[8]

In individual therapy, when therapists and patients both agree the woman is ready, she will need to go back to the unresolved childhood trauma that is driving her compulsivity. Family and childhood histories will provide clues as to how she became

This item has been checked out.

the way she is. Many of these women have complex PTSD from childhood abuse, witnessing abuse of others, and experiencing neglect, incest (overt or covert), or other sexual abuse. They also experience the consequences of addictive behaviors of other family members through reduced or excessive expectations or other mistreatment. For female sex offenders, punishment changes nothing and is all too familiar. Treatment must focus on the arrested development in childhood, the building of secure attachment bonds, trust, and choice to change the behavior.

One current, effective, and safe way to treat trauma is with emotional transformation therapy (ETT),[10] which combines primary colors, strobic lights, and peripheral eye stimulation to gently reflect to the patient what is going on inside. As she experiences her own system through engaging with the lights, along with coaching from the therapist, she learns about her attachment disorders, traumata, core beliefs, and areas of conflict.

A skilled ETT therapist can help patients modulate the intensity of the memory, using peripheral eye stimulation, to be more distant from the emotions while still able to experience and work through each emotion, body sensation, and distorted thinking. Dissociation can be diminished with colors and peripheral light. Shifts in cognition occur easily as emotions are experienced to completion, allowing a new perspective on the event. Through matching colors specific to body sensations, emotions, thoughts, and beliefs, and adjusting the intensity felt around the focus, patients experience release and are empowered to discover new insights. Regarding compulsive sexual behavior, ETT can help women discover the deficiencies behind their cravings to pursue sexual behaviors or drugs of choice. Key issues to explore are the parents' denial of a patient's reality, deprivation, abandonment, loneliness, and somatic complaints. When perspectives become those of an adult, emotions are manageable and new, more positive coping mechanisms will develop. The need for compulsive behaviors abates, as does the need for psychotropic medication.

Once trauma is resolved, therapy should emphasize developing appropriate social skills. Group therapy can be helpful with this phase, because a professional leader is present to coach and provide boundaries and safety. Most people want to be partnered, although some may choose celibacy. The goal is to be whole and know one's self as a sexual being, able to choose whether to be sexual with another. A greater capacity for intimacy and spirituality follow naturally.

One challenge of therapy is to reduce the pervasive shame and self-hatred; negative feelings and thoughts must be replaced with nurturing, playfulness, spiritual closeness, and meaningful communication. Robinson[11] suggests exercises for couples to help relationships last through promoting oxytocin (the bonding hormone) and downplaying dopamine-driven orgasms. These exercises are a useful way to structure interaction and learn parity in intimate relationships, while patients are still addressing their fear of closeness or relapse.

Below are illustrations of women in treatment for sexual compulsivity who bravely volunteered their stories to help other women and educate therapists. Their anonymity has been protected in this text.

CASE STUDIES OF WOMEN SUFFERING FROM SEXUAL COMPULSIVITY
Case 1: Woman Both Sexually Compulsive and Obsessed with Her Husband's Affairs

Joan is the middle child among three daughters. She was a beautiful but sensitive child who stuck closely by her mother's side. She was fearful of strangers and would scowl at them or refuse to smile. Her mother loved to dress her up and show her off. She was 5 years old when her father left to serve in the war. As a child Joan was terrified of her mother, whom she loved but was afraid would leave her. When her father left, however, she started sleeping with her mother, who would snuggle next to her "love child." It was then that Joan began a habit of rocking her hips. When her father returned she was bumped to another room.

Many years later, she asked her mother about her sexuality and was told her mother could have "automatic" orgasms in bed without a partner. Joan concluded she was unconsciously her mother's sexual partner. To this day she is not comfortable with the physical closeness of females. Joan considered herself a "bad seed" as a child. To complicate matters, her older sister tormented her.

Just before her father's return, Joan had her first sexual encounter with the girl next door, playing "genital games" in the closet of her parents' house. One day Joan was on the phone with this girl talking about their next sexual time together. Her mother overheard and told her to hang up but never said another word. Joan was mortified and really wanted to die. The absence of discussion made her feel worse.

Three years after her father's return, Joan began a physical relationship with the older sister who had tormented her. They would sleep on the third floor of the house and be orally sexual together. Her sister, who was 4 years older, used Joan to tease a boyfriend to meet them in the barn, or to play "spin the bottle" in the basement. Also during that time, a friend of her father molested Joan. When she told her mother, she was admonished never to tell her father or "he would kill the man." Joan was not allowed to express her feelings and remained fearful of this man, who lived down the street all through her adolescence. His daughter had previously been her best friend.

Masturbation fantasies (if Joan had time because of fears of being caught) were about sexual scenes she had witnessed with her sister and older cousins playing sexual games. Masturbation helped her relax and find pleasure in what was a very insecure and frightening world loaded with sexual energy. With her mother and sister exploiting her, she saw the world as out to get her. The only ally was her father, who was prone to depression. It was unfortunate that he was absent during her critical childhood years and then fairly unavailable after that because of work.

Her mother, meanwhile, continued her perpetration. She had all three of her daughters photographed nude at a clinic for child development as part of a study on growth patterns. She also had Joan model fashions as a young teen and always made a fuss over her hair. At one prom, Joan was forced to wear a gold dress and the hairstyle of Cleopatra. She came to feel that her body and soul did not belong to her.

Although her mother was a nurse and her father a doctor, no information about sexuality was imparted. Her mother seemed afraid of Joan's sexuality, yet did not protect Joan when others exploited her, although she would watch Joan like a hawk, threatening to tell her father if Joan were caught with a boy. The mother seemed obsessed with her daughters' respective sexualities (her older sister has been married three times and her younger sister was unfaithful to her husband). Joan was sexually abused on other occasions by older men and was also set up by her older sister for abuse by her college boyfriends; one of them French kissed her when she was 12 years old, which was traumatizing to her.

From the age of 10 years, Joan had a boyfriend in the neighborhood. They "petted" a lot but were never really sexual, being too scared and inexperienced. She had much longing for him, however, so they married when she was 19 and moved away from home to be in college together. She suspected her mother was involved in the plan to have her married. Joan did not adjust well in college (she also had dyslexia and attention deficit disorder), so she saw a school psychologist who told her she was a "cock teaser." Joan did not know what that term meant, but soon learned that men were attracted to her. Because Joan and her husband were not experienced and had no healthy sexual information, she concluded that they were incompatible. Their sex was fast, painful, and not at all romantic. She began having affairs, which she relates as the start of her sexual compulsion.

The affairs made her feel powerful and wanted. The first one was with a friend of her husband when she was 4 months pregnant. He soon learned of her husband's schedule and would visit when she was alone and seduce her. Their affair lasted until the baby was 6 months old. Her husband did not try to stop her even after reading a letter of passion from her to this man. One benefit from this affair was an improvement in sexual relations with her husband because she now knew more.

However, she also began to have one affair after another as she realized the immense power she had over the opposite sex. Most of the affairs were with the husbands of friends or teachers. She enjoyed the thrill of doing something secret. She was a wonderful lovely mother with many social skills, and in other places a powerful seductress who could have any man she wanted.

One man who was 10 years older taught her how to have an orgasm during intercourse. The next was the age of her parents and a famous teacher. She would visit her sister with her children and have sex with the men who also stayed at her sister's bed-and-breakfast. Joan experienced fun, excitement, and pleasure. She fell in love with a Latin musician (her father was also a musician) and decided to divorce her husband to be with him. However, it did not work out because he would not leave his wife. Her promiscuity increased to sleeping with different people all the time. She recalled feeling "crazy" as she took the 19-year-old cousin of a friend to bed, thinking it was his first time, which then made her feel like a predator.

Joan had three children before she left the marriage, experiencing much guilt around the impact of her behavior on her children and husband. After two more years of affairs, she fell in love again, but this time with another sexual compulsive. Both intended to stop the affairs by committing to each other. She married Dan but was unable to conceive. Dan wanted a child, so he had an affair with a woman who became pregnant. Joan felt so rejected by his affair that she retaliated with an emotional affair to palliate her feelings of worthlessness and emptiness. Dan continued having affairs, but Joan felt too much emotional pain to seek out anyone else, so she shifted to being obsessed with Dan's affairs. She compulsively searched for evidence of infidelity by examining his clothes, wallet, and briefcase. She would sit outside his office to see if he was still there. By this time, he was having affairs in his office, where he was also the boss. Joan was so devastated by Dan's affairs that she considered separation and divorce. At this time Joan agreed to go to a treatment program for sexual dependency. Dan sought treatment later.

Joan realized she was doing to him what she had done to her first husband. She saw that many of her behaviors were about rebellion and control, which she realized were reactions to her mother, whom she hated for setting her up for this aberrant sex life while trying to make sure she was not sexual before she married. Joan also thought her sister expected Joan to sleep with the men in her house. In being compulsively sexual, not only was there pleasure and excitement, but for once she was directing the whole thing by herself.

When Dan's last affair was discovered, Joan was distraught and felt foolish that she had trusted him yet again. Although they had both been attending 12-step meetings independently, they began to attend a Recovering Couples Anonymous (RCA) Twelve-Step Program, which added a third, vital dimension ("We") to their relationship. Through group support, Joan learned that women could be friends and that it is normal to have feelings and essential to have choices. She is learning to trust her intuition and not deny her reality. Joan is also beginning to communicate with Dan without shaming, blaming, or bringing up past hurts. Years later, she is forgiving herself for hurting others and is gaining an inner peace that benefits her on all levels. Her healing at a spiritual level has been significant. Dan and Joan have found richness in helping others, rather than rescuing them. They believe they have more intimacy and openness than most couples ever dream of having.

Comment

Joan was sexualized in childhood, perpetrated and controlled by her mother (a closet sexual compulsive who projected her disorder onto her daughters), and exploited by her older sister. She sought affairs for a sense of power and worth, which included exploiting others. Her second marriage was to another sexual compulsive, in which she continued the turbulent life she was groomed to live until she began treatment.

Case 2: Woman Alcoholic and Sexual Compulsive, Married to Man Who Overworked and Drank

Beth came from a family riddled with alcoholism and other abuses. Her father was charming, intelligent, and fluent in three languages, and graduated from college with top honors in 3 years. After his army assignment, he married her mother within 6 months of their meeting. His mean streak appeared soon after, which was worse when he was drunk.

As her father's drinking increased, he began to lose jobs. Her mother said he also had "strange ideas about sex." When Beth was 10 years old, her mother moved away with the children but did not keep her daughters from seeing their father. The father favored Beth because she was older and could learn things quickly. This situation gave her status but excluded her sister. She still feels guilt toward her sister, who is practically homeless from addictions and poor choices and who neglected her son, whom Beth is raising.

Father showed Beth sexual photographs when she was young. She also remembers feeling confused and anxious when he said things like "don't be a cockteaser," that her mother was "not very good in bed," and "if I were 20 years younger, and you were not my daughter…" He showed her "how boys pee" when she was only 5 years old. Beth received no education about sex except from a book at puberty. Sex was never discussed at home. In fourth grade, after her parents' divorce, an adult male "friend" shared his pornography with Beth and masturbated in front of her, telling her he could not help himself because she was so pretty. He said he knew he could trust her not to tell anyone. When Beth was 16 years old, he stalked her and then molested her in a tent.

Her first intense relationship started in adolescence and lasted 6 years. She and her lover began sexual relations when she was 16 years old. They often fought and neither was faithful. When drinking, Beth was very sexual and had many partners. This activity stayed hidden. In public, she was a perfect girl, class scholar, and athlete.

Soon after graduation from college, Beth met Jerry, to whom she became engaged. In her wisdom she saw him as a man of integrity, steady, and stable in his life, unlike her family's male role models. They had an "amazing courtship," being madly in love on all levels, but their relationship also involved drinking and drugging. Jerry was a compulsive worker, which allowed Beth to function independently, including raising the children and having affairs.

They had great family vacations, but otherwise Jerry worked all the time. They both drank a lot, but Jerry began to have episodes of drunkenness, which were upsetting to Beth. He attended Alcoholics Anonymous (AA) meetings and eventually stopped drinking entirely for 16 years. The compulsive working continued, however. Beth began to drink more heavily herself, and started going out with friends without him. Feeling estranged, Jerry began to drink again so he could rejoin her.

Beth stopped her drinking and affairs 3 years ago, after Jerry discovered her having sex with a neighbor in their basement. Jerry was devastated and unable to function; Beth was the greatest love of his life and caused him the worst pain. He became severely depressed. Beth went to treatment and now his drinking makes her uncomfortable again, but she can address it with him. The truth slowly emerged about her affairs and childhood abuse. Beth has been sober from alcohol and has abstained sex outside the marriage since that time. Jerry began therapy and is beginning to understand how his childhood situation contributed to his excessive sense of responsibility and neglect of his marriage and children. Both have received ongoing help through individual, couple, and group psychotherapy, along with 12-step meetings.

Beth and Jerry realize that they need to spend much more time just talking and doing things together to maintain their love and understanding. It is easy to disengage unintentionally while raising children and overscheduling. They also realize the importance of a support system to help them address difficult topics. These challenges are ongoing.

Comment

Beth was sexualized by her father and insufficiently protected by her mother, and experienced the impact of generations of alcoholism. Her parents divorced and a family friend sexually abused her, after which she became sexually active and promiscuous. She married a man who remained oblivious to her behavior because of his drinking, taking drugs, and working compulsively. This situation allowed her to resume having affairs until her behavior was finally discovered and she was sent to treatment.

Case 3: Divorced Woman with One Child

Susan originally sought treatment for her alcoholism. A year into treatment, she cautiously admitted she had another addiction: sexual compulsivity. She had a good job with a corporation, but was promiscuous in her private life or when traveling. Her family of origin was Catholic and was considered the "church family" because priests and nuns liked to visit. Their house was fairly isolated, located on a farm, and had a pool. Her family life was characterized by alcoholism, fighting, inappropriate behavior, and neglect of the children. Susan was molested by the farm hands. She discovered masturbation at 3 years of age and used it to cope. She was also sexual with the pet dog. In school she was outgoing and popular.

As a young adult, she worked as an exotic dancer by night and became indiscriminate about sexual partners. By day she had a corporate job and was moving up the ladder. After work, drinking and smoking were also part of her scene. She became pregnant from one encounter and had a child. She married the father, who was soon sent to jail for committing a crime. Susan divorced and raised the child alone, sometimes bringing men home for sex. Her disease progressed dangerously until she was participating in snuff movies (movies in which participants are actually abused and die).

Fortunately, some healthy part of her knew this behavior could result in death, so she stopped and began looking for help. She first attended AA and then meetings for sexual compulsivity and group and individual therapy. She chose celibacy and gained weight, but avoided the sexual compulsivity for many years, helping others to recover by offering workshops and running groups for recovering sexual compulsives. She then learned she had uterine cancer, from which she died—an unfortunate probable consequence of her disease.

Comment

Susan experienced PTSD, came from an alcoholic family, was neglected and sexually abused in childhood, and acted out her trauma in the "Looking for Mr. Goodbar" style. In recovery, she transformed her experience into a gift of helping others. She remained celibate, protected partially by her obesity, and never established another intimate relationship with a partner.

Case 4: Celibate, Codependent, Alcoholic Woman with Sexual Compulsivity and Compulsive Attitudes Toward Food and Spending

Amy grew up in housing projects for the poor. When her mother was in the hospital giving birth to Amy, her father was in bed with another woman. The family had little money because her parents both drank and partied. Home life was characterized by violence, physical abuse, and neglect. She does not recall her mother ever changing the sheets or telling them to take a bath. The children grew up eating sodas and pretzels. Her mother would cook dinner, but if it was not perfect the father would rage and throw the dishes. If any of the four daughters laughed, she was hit.

Sometimes her father would be so drunk he would urinate while passed out on the sofa, in bed, or wherever he fell down. Amy would have to fetch him from the bars to come home for dinner. No breakfast was served and noise was not allowed because her mother was always hung-over from drinking.

Around Amy's fourth birthday, her mother lost twins who were only one week old. Her mother never recovered from that loss despite having another daughter a few years later, so Amy's birthday was consistently overlooked. Only at Christmas did Amy feel cared about because she received lots of presents that included things they needed. The best times were those she spent with her grandmother, who cooked breakfast, bought her clothes, and put her to bed in clean sheets and pajamas. Amy wet the bed at home but never at her grandmother's house.

As a child, Amy also liked to play with matches and once set the sofa on fire in the same room where her mother was playing cards. Her mother also would awaken the children any time of night to play cards or make them punch her fist to show their strength. She slapped, pinched, and hit her children if she thought they lied or did things that might look bad to the neighbors. Amy was not allowed to leave the block on which they lived until she was 15 years old. Amy learned early to dissociate when she was beaten so she could just wait it out; from early childhood, she did not cry or show anger.

Because she believed herself stupid and worthless, Amy seldom studied for school and therefore did not do well (another reason for her mother to hit her) unless encouraged by a teacher who took an interest in her. She enjoyed sports and liked to draw, which were her strengths. As an adolescent, she began drinking and going to parties where she would drink to get drunk. She continued to play several sports well, and being "one of the guys" in sports became her identity and a protection from dating and abuse. She also learned to be enterprising in ways to earn money, even stealing, to keep the family going. By tenth grade, she had several jobs so she could buy cigarettes, clothes, and alcohol. She also borrowed, and stole, money from her mother. When she received her paychecks Amy had to repay her mother, leaving little for herself. The cycle continued because Amy could not become physically or financially independent of her family.

Amy's sexual activity began when she discovered masturbation at 4 years of age while playing with a hangar with a friend. Rubbing the hanger against her genitals created a new pleasurable sensation. She used it to relax and put herself to sleep and to escape the unpredictable and chaotic life of her family. Soon she did not need the hanger and would hide in a closet to masturbate. She found that masturbation helped her with all of her uncomfortable feelings and became her main coping mechanism for the next 44 years. She would try to engage her sister in kissing as a way to be sexual, but her mother caught them and said people would think they were gay. Next she tried to find a way to be touched genitally by playing card games, like strip poker, and would intentionally lose. She went to her first X-rated movie at 16 years of age. She also peeped through cracks in the wall of a men's locker room to watch them walk around after taking a shower.

By 19 years of age, Amy began hanging out with a friend instead of at the playground. They learned about a program that allowed them to teach sports and go to school. Her friend was accepted, and although Amy believed herself too stupid to be accepted, she got a job teaching sports to children. She believed she had found the ideal situation. She and her friend taught together, drank, and partied. She continued living at home and being abused by her mother for another 2 years. It did not occur to her to move out or tell her mother to stop. Her job was to fix the family.

As an adult, Amy had no sexual relationships but did have some dates. She was unaware that she dissociated during these dates until one guy gently told her he would not hurt her. Because Amy feared men and becoming pregnant, she decided to try sex with women. She tried to seduce her friend but became afraid of the intimacy and stopped. Her friend did not understand and felt hurt. Amy had an active fantasy life (which always included a violent component) to which she masturbated. She does not recall sexual abuse as a child, but the physical abuse became eroticized.

Amy then joined a convent, which enabled her to go to college and study to become a teacher. She chose celibacy because she feared that if she had children she might abuse them. She also hoped she would feel safe and have a chance for a better life as a nun. At college, however, one of her teachers molested her and another was inappropriate. Because of her habit of suppressing feelings in childhood to survive, she never protested. As a nun, she dedicated her life to helping her family and others, treating everyone equally and never allowing herself to be angry or even defend herself. She would occasionally feel resentful about being taken advantage of and having no time for herself. Masturbation, computer games, alcohol, and food extinguished those feelings.

To make her addiction to alcohol less obvious, Amy tried to control her drinking, but it did not really work. After she was told to stop drinking or leave the convent, she stopped for 2 years. However, when her mother was dying and no one in the family would help, Amy went home to care for her. Because she could not bear the pain of watching her mother deteriorate and seeing her father beat her when she couldn't keep doing the things he wanted, Amy experienced a relapse. Her mother's death meant the loss of any opportunity to experience her love.

Because Amy did not feel supported where she lived she continued to drink. By now, however, she had taken final vows and could not be forced to leave. She developed a huge breast abscess requiring surgical treatment. Being very depressed, she was also sent to a psychiatrist and spiritual director, and then to inpatient treatment for 12 months and aftercare for several years. During that time, her father and grandfather died, and her support system helped prevent her from a relapse. Still, she resisted opening up fully about her sexual compulsivity. She kept flirting at AA meetings for a rush, but never went further. Eventually she addressed her sexual compulsivity, with resistance but much courage.

Treatment has been slow, as expected. Because of the trauma, her trust is limited and emotions are still frightening. Amy feels nauseous or dissociates when the emotions emerge. ETT peripheral light stimulation has enabled her to break down emotions into small components so she can tolerate them and stay focused in therapy; she is now more present than ever before. When her throat clogs, looking at the color blue helps her clear it and find her voice. If Amy looks at the chart of primary colors and her feelings approach the threshold at which she begins dissociating, the colors all fade out. When she can tolerate the colors peripherally, they all come back. This effect amazes her and has decreased her fear of her feelings.

Amy attends a therapy group for abused women, a spiritual direction group, and regular 12-step meetings, plus she receives Reiki treatments. She still has difficulty saying "no" to helping her family and others, but is slowly finding time to paint and golf. Spending other people's money, eating junk food, and giving too much of herself away are issues that still require attention. She has been sober from sexual compulsivity for several years and from alcohol for 12 years. She is much more present and is beginning to let people get to know her a little, although she still wants to do things for them to earn their friendship. Years of diligence with a strong recovery program and support system have helped her achieve a self-actualization she could not have otherwise imagined.

Comment

Amy experienced serious deprivation, neglect, and abuse in childhood, resulting in PTSD. Her mother was unable to nurture or bond in a consistent way, creating an avoidant attachment disorder in Amy. Her father was playful only when drunk, but also mostly violent. His violence conditioned her to be so terrified of men that she has never sought a sexual experience. She chose celibacy to prevent passing on child abuse.

She masturbated from early childhood to save her sanity, incorporating the violence she witnessed into her fantasies. Her sexual compulsivity was harder to give up than alcohol. Spunk, sports, creativity, and resourcefulness have been important assets to her recovery.

Case 5: Unmarried Woman with Sexual Anorexia after Years of Compulsive Sexuality and Stable but Unresolved Posttraumatic Stress Disorder from Childhood

Pam is the oldest of three children to parents who raised her to be a "trophy child." They were overly protective and would not let her date or make independent choices. They made her attend classes to find a future husband. Her father was verbally abusive to her and sexualized her without touching her. When she asked why he kept staring at her, he replied that she was so beautiful. He was a violent man and she was terrified of him, yet felt like his mistress. She felt hated and reviled by him "like a cigarette stub." Her mother was also verbally abused by the father and would complain about him to Pam during the day but not defend or protect Pam from him when he came home. She never had a champion. Her mother never took enough interest in her to teach social skills, hygiene, or how to dress. Girls teased her for her dirty nails and scuffed shoes. When the father came home from work, her mother stayed silent but drank to the point of passing out. The house was filthy from neglect. Pam kept her own room very clean and decided that she had to raise herself.

From an early age, she knew she did not want marriage or children. By 9 years of age, Pam was chubby. By 13 years, she was anorexic (with food) and then later bulimic. She began to dress provocatively and sneak out of the house to date, but was "deathly afraid of sex." She had been on the honor roll in school, but once her sexual behavior escalated she flunked classes and then quit school to pursue sexual conquests.

Pam moved out of the house at 18 years of age and never returned. She grew up hating men, using them for sex only. She also avoided women as friends, fearing they would reject her. She chose men who were socially beneath her, believing they would not reject her, yet she tolerated their using and dumping her. She loved clothes. At one time she said she had 50 pairs of high heels all with their own polish. Her house had an entire room dedicated to sex toys and bondage. She feels "held and loved" in bondage. Fortunately, she said she's had no sexually transmitted diseases, although she developed reflex sympathetic dystrophy, which has been painful and limits her activities.

In 1990, she found her way to 12-step meetings for sexual compulsives and stopped the behavior, choosing to become sexually anorexic. She continued to dress provocatively, however, and became angry if this was mentioned in the meetings. Eventually she stopped going to the meetings, because the stories were too painful to hear and too many men were present. She said she always put on a happy face but felt "rotten, defective, and unlovable" inside.

She lives an isolated life, not able to trust anyone and fearing relapse into compulsive sexuality. Prozac helped stop her promiscuity. She has had a few sexual slips but manages to return to celibacy. She would like to have sex once in a while without having to deal with a relationship. Her ideal man is blond, muscular, and 25 years of age. Pam is now in her 50s. She has had facelifts, bleaches her hair, and uses make-up to maintain her good looks. She experiences depression, loneliness, and obsessive negative thoughts. Zoloft, neurontin, and buspar have helped stabilize her considerably.

Pam relates to animals more than people, has many pets, especially cats, and donates up to $24,000 a year to shelters and charities for animals. In the past few years she became a vegetarian, considering it a triumph for the animals. For a while she made and sold dried and silk flower arrangements and gave the profits to animal causes. She was successful and learned a lot, but the arrangements became too labor-intensive for too little profit. Her parents supported her in this endeavor, and her father finally gave Pam her own checking account. He had previously given her a house and trust fund. Pam believes he finally realized he ruined her for relationships. She is grateful for this financial security.

Pam has other compulsive behaviors, such as cleaning, weight-lifting, food, shopping for clothes, speeding, and going to concerts. She is able to put the brakes on these for the most part, and hopes God will forgive her for being promiscuous. She has much remorse for her behaviors and believes she must do more service on this planet to earn her place in Heaven. She has considered counseling other women but tends to assume their pain, as she did her mother's, and then feels responsible. She occasionally has suicidal ideation, but, again wanting the mercy of God, tries to be good. Her father died a couple of years ago. Pam felt relief, but anger still lies just beneath the surface. She said she still acts out the sex kitten role that her father groomed her for, only now she empowers herself with choices. Her mother has a new lease on life without the father. She gives Pam money to compensate for having abandoned her in childhood. Pam also sees it as hush money.

Comment

Pam experienced covert sexual abuse, sexual anorexia, and PTSD with an avoidant attachment disorder. She was sexualized by her violent, possessive and oppressive father and not protected by her alcoholic, avoidant mother. She is unable to feel comfortable with people and lacks the social skills to thrive in American culture, and therefore remains isolated and lonely. She is too fragile to perform trauma work but accepts medication. She trusts animals more than people and crusades for them. Sadly, this is probably as far as she can go in recovery.

SUMMARY

This article discusses women who have sexual compulsivity, a disorder that is intensely shame-based and difficult to treat. The case studies presented show the family preconditioning of abandonment in childhood through inadequate care, abuse, neglect, and the presence of other addictions. As children, these women searched for something to soothe their distress when they could not rely on their caregivers. Maladaptive coping mechanisms, such as masturbation, food, romantic or violent fantasies, and any behavior to would gain attention, maintained their sanity in childhood. However, these behaviors also advanced to autonomy, eliminating the option of choices. In adulthood, the numbing of psychic pain by these found solutions became a preoccupation around which life was organized. Consequences developed and as the disease progressed, large amounts of time were regularly lost in fantasy and ritualistic behaviors, causing life to become unmanageable. The fear of being discovered, loneliness, and sexually transmitted diseases typically escalates to spiritual bankruptcy and eventual spiritual, psychological, and possibly physical death. The dilemma is too deep and powerful for women to heal themselves over time, partly because of her impaired thinking, unresolved trauma, and desperation-driven repeat of the behaviors. Proper intervention and treatment can make a difference.

Restoration to full health takes years, requiring diligence, motivation, and a therapist who is knowledgeable, committed, patient, and willing to use all available modalities. Trust is a huge issue for these women, and even when taking a positive risk in therapy, trauma responses from early childhood may be evoked. These women are exquisitely sensitive to criticism, but if feeling safe most can learn to trust and will respond to help, because they long to be restored to their values, be self-sufficient, and have a voice that is respected. Uncovering sexual secrets from previous generations, still present in the families-of-origin, helps patients put their problems in context. Treatment can be successful if patients develop a capacity to bond, can tolerate the psychic pain of disclosure, are willing to be accountable, are resilient, and can forgive themselves and others. The rewards for this endeavor are great. The successful interruption and healing of patterns of abuse, shame, and distortions of intimacy and sexuality is a great contribution to society.

RESEARCH AND FUTURE DEVELOPMENT

The Society for the Advancement of Sexual Health (SASH) addresses sex compulsivity. SASH has an excellent journal dedicated to this topic, *The Journal of Sexual Addiction and Compulsivity*, published quarterly by Taylor and Francis.[10] A helpful and highly recommended supplement to this article, entitled "Women and Sexual Addiction," was published in a 2002 issue of the journal.[4]

Despite the growing prevalence of sexual compulsivity, the general public does not embrace the concept of disordered sexuality, partly because the sex industry generates billions of dollars in revenues each year. Persons experiencing sexual compulsivity, such as those in the presented cases, have been the real pioneers in reaching out for help and teaching professionals about their personal experience. They deserve help not only for their own pain but also to advance sexual health in American culture that will lead to better treatment of children in the future. Lessons about healthy courtship and proper parenting should also be required in educational institutions for all children and adults.

REFERENCES

1. Carnes P. Out of the shadows: understanding sexual addiction. 3rd edition. Center City (MN): Hazelden; 2001.

2. Carnes P. Don't call it love: recovery from sexual addiction. New York: Bantam Books; 1991.
3. Carnes P, Delmonico D, Griffin E. In the shadows of the net: breaking free of compulsive online sexual behavior. Center City (MN): Hazelden; 2001.
4. Cooper A, Delmonico D, Burg R. Cybersex users, abusers, and compulsives: the dark side of the force. Journal of Sexual Addiction and Compulsivity 2000;7(1–2): 5–30.
5. Rossner Judith. Looking for Mr. Goodbar. London: Coronet Books; 1977.
6. Kasl CD. Women, sex, and addiction: a search for love and power. New York: Ticknor & Fields; 1989.
7. Rutter P. Sex, power and boundaries: understanding and preventing sexual harassments. New York: Bantam Books; 1996.
8. Kasl CD. Many roads, one journey: moving beyond the twelve Steps. New York: Harper Perennial; 1992.
9. Bear E, editor. Female sexual abusers: three views (Davin, Hislop and Dunbar). Brandon (VT): Safer Society Press; 1999.
10. Vazquez S. A new paradigm for PTSD treatment: emotional transformation therapy. Annals of the American Psychotherapy Association 2005;Summer:18–25.
11. Robinson M. Peace between the sheets: healing with sexual relationships. Berkeley (CA): Frog Ltd; 2004.

Index

Note: Page numbers of article titles are in **boldface** type.

A

Addiction, in compulsive cybersex behavior, 704–705
    in persons with compulsive sexual behavior, 608
    out-of-control sexual behavior as, 598
Addictive cycles, 582-583, 704–705
Affect dysregulation, in abused children, 574
Affectional systems, developmental model of, 572
Affect suppression, as sexuality, 575
Attachment, and self systems, 572–574
    avoidant, 570-571, 574–575
    disorganized, 571, 572–573, 662
    impaired sense of self and, 569–571
    insecure, 661–662
    in sexually compulsive adolescents, 661–662
    patterns of, 570–571
    secure, 570, 661–662
    sexually compulsive behavior and, 569–575
Attachment disorder, paraphilias and, 675–677
Attachment trauma, in sexually compulsive adolescents, 661–662
      therapies for, 664–666

C

Child abuse and neglect, sexual behavior and, 572
Childhood sexual abuse, as risk factor for compulsive sexual behavior, 609
    compulsive sexual behavior and, 609
Childhood sexual abuse victim, as dissociated sex offender, 600–601
    as victimizer, 577
    bottoming out of, 579
    trauma re-enactments by, 575, 578
Children, sexualized, 582
    sexually abused, 572–578
Cognitive-behavioral therapy (CBT), for compulsive cybersex behavior, 706
    for sexually compulsive adolescents, 663
Cognitive-behavioral therapy with relapse prevention component (CBT/RP), in sexual
    offender treatment, 681–682
Compulsive cybersex behavior, addiction cycle in, 704–705
    case studies, Anne: compulsive self-treatment of anger, stress, depression, 701–703
      Dan: obsession in hair-cutting fetish reenactment of childhood sexual abuse,
        700–701

Psychiatr Clin N Am 31 (2008) 729–737
doi:10.1016/S0193-953X(08)00094-4
0193-953X/08/$ – see front matter © 2008 Elsevier Inc. All rights reserved.

psych.theclinics.com

United States Postal Service

Statement of Ownership, Management, and Circulation
(All Periodicals Publications Except Requestor Publications)

1. Publication Title	2. Publication Number	3. Filing Date
Psychiatric Clinics of North America	0 0 0 − 7 0 3	9/15/08

4. Issue Frequency	5. Number of Issues Published Annually	6. Annual Subscription Price
Mar, Jun, Sep, Dec	4	$213.00

7. Complete Mailing Address of Known Office of Publication (Not printer) (Street, city, county, state, and ZIP+4)

Elsevier Inc.
360 Park Avenue South
New York, NY 10010-1710

Contact Person
Stephen Bushing

Telephone (Include area code)
215-239-3688

8. Complete Mailing Address of Headquarters or General Business Office of Publisher (Not printer)

Elsevier Inc., 360 Park Avenue South, New York, NY 10010-1710

9. Full Names and Complete Mailing Addresses of Publisher, Editor, and Managing Editor (Do not leave blank)

Publisher (Name and complete mailing address)

John Schrefer, Elsevier, Inc., 1600 John F. Kennedy Blvd. Suite 1800, Philadelphia, PA 19103-2899

Editor (Name and complete mailing address)

Sarah Barth, Elsevier, Inc., 1600 John F. Kennedy Blvd. Suite 1800, Philadelphia, PA 19103-2899

Managing Editor (Name and complete mailing address)

Catherine Bewick, Elsevier, Inc., 1600 John F. Kennedy Blvd. Suite 1800, Philadelphia, PA 19103-2899

10. Owner (Do not leave blank. If the publication is owned by a corporation, give the name and address of the corporation immediately followed by the names and addresses of all stockholders owning or holding 1 percent or more of the total amount of stock. If not owned by a corporation, give the names and addresses of the individual owners. If owned by a partnership or other unincorporated firm, give its name and address as well as those of each individual owner. If the publication is published by a nonprofit organization, give its name and address.)

Full Name	Complete Mailing Address
Wholly owned subsidiary of	4520 East-West Highway
Reed/Elsevier, US holdings	Bethesda, MD 20814

11. Known Bondholders, Mortgagees, and Other Security Holders Owning or Holding 1 Percent or More of Total Amount of Bonds, Mortgages, or Other Securities. If none, check box. ☐ None

Full Name	Complete Mailing Address
N/A	

12. Tax Status (For completion by nonprofit organizations authorized to mail at nonprofit rates) (Check one)
The purpose, function, and nonprofit status of this organization and the exempt status for federal income tax purposes:
☐ Has Not Changed During Preceding 12 Months
☐ Has Changed During Preceding 12 Months (Publisher must submit explanation of change with this statement)

PS Form 3526, September 2006 (Page 1 of 3 (Instructions Page 3)) PSN 7530-01-000-9931 PRIVACY NOTICE: See our Privacy policy in www.usps.com

13. Publication Title	14. Issue Date for Circulation Data Below
Psychiatric Clinics of North America	September 2008

15. Extent and Nature of Circulation		Average No. Copies Each Issue During Preceding 12 Months	No. Copies of Single Issue Published Nearest to Filing Date
a. Total Number of Copies (Net press run)		2100	2000
b. Paid Circulation (By Mail and Outside the Mail)	(1) Mailed Outside-County Paid Subscriptions Stated on PS Form 3541. (Include paid distribution above nominal rate, advertiser's proof copies, and exchange copies)	1082	1016
	(2) Mailed In-County Paid Subscriptions Stated on PS Form 3541 (Include paid distribution above nominal rate, advertiser's proof copies, and exchange copies)		
	(3) Paid Distribution Outside the Mails Including Sales Through Dealers and Carriers, Street Vendors, Counter Sales, and Other Paid Distribution Outside USPS®	356	339
	(4) Paid Distribution by Other Classes Mailed Through the USPS (e.g. First-Class Mail®)		
c. Total Paid Distribution (Sum of 15b (1), (2), (3), and (4))	▶	1438	1355
d. Free or Nominal Rate Distribution (By Mail and Outside the Mail)	(1) Free or Nominal Rate Outside-County Copies Included on PS Form 3541	77	76
	(2) Free or Nominal Rate In-County Copies Included on PS Form 3541		
	(3) Free or Nominal Rate Copies Mailed at Other Classes Mailed Through the USPS (e.g. First-Class Mail)		
	(4) Free or Nominal Rate Distribution Outside the Mail (Carriers or other means)		
e. Total Free or Nominal Rate Distribution (Sum of 15d (1), (2), (3) and (4))	▶	77	76
f. Total Distribution (Sum of 15c and 15e)	▶	1515	1431
g. Copies not Distributed (See instructions to publishers #4 (page #3))	▶	585	569
h. Total (Sum of 15f and g)	▶	2100	2000
i. Percent Paid (15c divided by 15f times 100)		94.92%	94.69%

16. Publication of Statement of Ownership

☐ If the publication is a general publication, publication of this statement is required. Will be printed in the December 2008 issue of this publication.   ☐ Publication not required

17. Signature and Title of Editor, Publisher, Business Manager, or Owner

[signature]

John Famacci – Executive Director of Subscription Services

Date
September 15, 2008

I certify that all information furnished on this form is true and complete. I understand that anyone who furnishes false or misleading information on this form or who omits material or information requested on the form may be subject to criminal sanctions (including fines and imprisonment) and/or civil sanctions (including civil penalties).

PS Form 3526, September 2006 (Page 2 of 3)